Praise

First Do No

"A succinct and thorough analysis of the current challenges and myths of the Canadian health care system...Canadians interested in health care will want to read it...health care providers, planners, and politicians must read it!"

PHILIP ELLISON, MD, MBA, CCFP, FCFP, DOHS
ACTING CHAIR, DEPARTMENT OF FAMILY AND COMMUNITY MEDICINE
UNIVERSITY OF TORONTO
FAMILY PHYSICIAN-IN-CHIEF
UNIVERSITY HEALTH NETWORK

➤

"*First Do No Harm* is a superb brief description of Canada's health care system—its strengths and its problems. Readable and informative, it will be a valuable guide for Canadians who want to understand the critical health care policy choices their country is facing. Americans, too, will find this book absorbing and instructive. It is a gem.

ARNOLD S. RELMAN, M.D.
PROFESSOR OF MEDICINE AND SOCIAL MEDICINE, HARVARD MEDICAL SCHOOL
EDITOR-IN-CHIEF EMERITUS, *NEW ENGLAND JOURNAL OF MEDICINE*

➤

"...*First Do No Harm* offers compelling dialogue on how to master sensible reforms for our national health system. The book reinforces home care's vital role in improving the system's effectiveness...and the fundamental need to establish a national approach to home care to support this role."

SHIRLEE SHARKEY
PRESIDENT & CEO, SAINT ELIZABETH HEALTH CARE, AND CURRENT PRESIDENT,
REGISTERED NURSES ASSOCIATION OF ONTARIO

➤

"...the health care debate reflects, in part...[the] issue of creating and sustaining tolerant, socially just societies in the 21st century...[and the need] to 'fight' a possible slide and keep a democratic, socially just society in Canada. *First Do No Harm*, although it is about health care, is, in my view, also about this broader issue."

FRASER MUSTARD
THE CANADIAN INSTITUTE FOR ADVANCED RESEARCH

➤

"Finally—a 'primer' to help ordinary Canadians understand just what the health care debate is really all about...and the complex challenges we face in fixing the genuine shortcomings without destroying the very real benefits."

WENDY L. ARMSTRONG
PAST PRESIDENT
HEALTH COMMITTEE OF ALBERTA CONSUMERS' ASSOCIATION

FIRST DO NO HARM

MAKING SENSE OF CANADIAN HEALTH REFORM

TERRENCE SULLIVAN

PATRICIA M. BARANEK

WITH

MALCOLM ANDERSON, TOM ARCHIBALD,
MORRIS BARER, PETER COYTE, RAISA DEBER,
COLLEEN FLOOD, STEVEN LEWIS,
KAREN PARENT, AND SAM SHORTT

UBCPress · Vancouver · Toronto

Originally published in 2002 by Malcolm Lester and Associates, Toronto, Ontario.
Reprinted in 2003 by UBC Press.

09 08 07 06 05 04 03   5 4 3 2

Printed in Canada on acid-free paper ∞

National Library of Canada Cataloguing in Publication Data

Sullivan, Terrence James, 1951-
    First do no harm: making sense of Canadian health reform /
    Terrence Sullivan, Patricia M. Baranek

Includes bibliographical references and index.
ISBN 0-7748-1016-5

I. Health care reform – Canada. I. Baranek, Patricia M., 1946- II. Title.

RA395.C3S92 2002   362.1'0971   C2002-911168-4

Canadä

UBC Press gratefully acknowledges the financial support for our publishing
program of the Government of Canada through the Book Publishing Industry
Development Program (BPIDP), and of the Canada Council for the Arts, and
the British Columbia Arts Council.

This book has been published with the help of a grant from the Humanities and
Social Sciences Federation of Canada, using funds provided by the Social Sciences
and Humanities Research Council of Canada.

Book design: Jack Steiner

UBC Press
The University of British Columbia
2029 West Mall
Vancouver, BC V6T 1Z2
604-822-5959 / Fax: 604-822-6083
www.ubcpress.ca

For Megan, Jesse, Sarah, Kate, and Joshua—Canada's children,
that they may inherit a high-quality health care system
as a privilege of citizenship

➤

The physician must be able to tell the antecedents, know the present, and foretell the future, must mediate these things, and have two special objects in view with regard to disease, namely to do good or to do no harm.

HIPPOCRATES, *OF THE EPIDEMICS*, 400 BC,
TRANSLATED BY FRANCIS ADAMS

CONTENTS

This is a very important little book indeed! It is about looking at our health care system from unusual angles—an exercise in itself stimulating and enriching—but, above all, it is about clarifying words and facts, and about initiating discussion about the future of medicare.

Canadians are proud of their health care system; even as they worry about its future, it remains—as it has for decades—the most loved social program in the country. Only 30 years old, medicare has become deeply entrenched in the Canadian identity. But it has also become a very emotional issue; so much so that what was meant to simply be a legislative tool to correct extra-billing and user fees— the Canada Health Act (1984)—has become an icon. The five criteria or conditions of the legislation have become the five principles of our health care system. When Canada was named the best country in the world to live in, medicare was a significant part of that achievement. I understand the emotions surrounding the issue. Politics and public policies are, after all, about values. And values are neither neutral nor objective. They are about commitment.

The Romanow Commission is now giving us a unique opportunity to pause, to discuss—not to fight for or against a cause, however good—and to assess what exactly we want medicare to become, at what cost, and under what conditions. Canada's health care system is no longer a simple program that offers "free" hospital services and doctors' care. Its organizational dimensions are complex, as are its financing, its delivery, and its various institutional cultures. So, to discuss it intelligently, to "make sense" of it, we need a common understanding of what we are talking about and on what we base our thinking.

That is what this book does. *First Do No Harm* informs, explains, dispels preconceived ideas, debunks myths, and explodes dogmas. It offers a remarkably clear, concise, and comprehensive picture of our health care system. Above all, it always uses *le mot juste*. No compromise is allowed here!

Terry Sullivan and Pat Baranek take us through the generalizations we hear repeatedly—at home and south of the border—about what is wrong with the way we provide health care and what the remedies are. They present the evidence and spell out the arguments, but they are not doctrinaire. They establish the facts about health care spending and about its financing. They clarify what is public and what is private—a key dimension for discussion right now. They discuss user fees, waiting lists, and privatization. They touch on some of the recent "best practices" initiatives. Home care, national standards, and pharmacare are all part of Sullivan and Baranek's dialogue. And finally, they invite us to think "outside of the box" about the future of health care in Canada.

As a bonus, this very well-informed, evidence-based, integrated discussion of our health care system is lively and reads easily. The book was written out of the authors' love of learning and we all benefit from it.

THE HON. MONIQUE BÉGIN, PC

Monique Bégin is former Minister of Health for Canada and former Dean of Health Sciences at the University of Ottawa. She still teaches in the University of Ottawa's Health Administration Program.

Contrary to popular belief, the traditional medical imperative—
Primum non nocere or "First Do No Harm"—is not to be found, as
commonly thought, in the Hippocratic oath, but the equivalent
phrase does appear in *Of The Epidemics* by Hippocrates.

There are many reforms required in Canada's health care system and, as we write this volume, the Romanow Commission on the
Future of Health Care in Canada is hearing the full range of ideas.
These reforms, in our view, should be approached with the same
care, concern, and informed judgement—based on evidence and
real life experience—with which the best physicians approach the
care of ill patients. Many simple solutions from other fields, when
applied to our health care problems, do not withstand the hard
scrutiny of international and domestic evidence and experience.

About three years ago, in spite of comprehensive advice from
the National Forum on Health and in the face of rising concern
about health care in this country, the government of Canada took
little action on health reform. The Atkinson Foundation convened
a small group of leaders in the health sector, including a number of
academics, health economists, and officials, to reflect on this problem and provoke public debate on some fundamental issues facing
a reform agenda. A steering committee was then established, com-
posed of Monique Bégin, Peter Coyte, Michael Decter, Colleen
Flood, Vivek Goel, Doris Grinspun, Steven Lewis, Jim Maclean, Tom
Noseworthy, and Greg Stoddard, chaired by Terrence Sullivan with
analytic and organizational support and full participation from
Patricia Baranek. With their assistance and advice, the Dialogue on
Health Reform was launched.

With financial support from the Atkinson Foundation, the working group commissioned papers on a limited number of topical
issues that were of strategic importance to the health reform
debate:[1] papers on health financing (Raisa B. Deber), waiting lists
(Sam Shortt, Morris Barer, and Steven Lewis), home care (Peter
Coyte, Malcolm Anderson, and Karen Parent), legal constraints on
private medicine (Colleen Flood and Tom Archibald). Much of the
material in this book is drawn from these papers. Though we have

taken their original work as the main underpinning of this volume, these authors are in no way responsible for any error on our part in presenting or interpreting their work.

The organization of the volume follows the spirit and logic of the background papers. In the first chapter we identify some key features of health care arrangements in Canada, which, in our view, are worth preserving in some fashion. We also identify areas in need of change. We review the range of concerns about health care in Canada and how these concerns have changed over time, how they compare with other jurisdictions, and what features of our system are worth considering as important benchmarks for any reform plans we might undertake. In Chapter 2, we explore the financing of our system and the interplay of federal and provincial roles and jurisdictions in this financing. Chapter 3 expressly takes on a number of common myths about health care in Canada and tries to explore how these stack up against evidence from here and elsewhere. Chapter 4 deals with the challenging and vexatious problem of reducing waiting times and waiting lines in Canada. Chapter 5 lays out what we know about home care arrangements and the reform options for creating national standards in this expanding site of care. Chapter 6 sketches out three possible scenarios for reform and checks them against the features we identified in the first chapter.

The volume is not a comprehensive approach to reform issues, but a topical commentary on some of the more common, challenging and frequently muddled ideas that are in the public discussion on health reform in Canada. We offer these ideas in the hope that they may prove useful and informative to interested citizens as we rethink how best to reform and revitalize our health care system. If the hallmarks of tolerant, prosperous societies are a productive economy and distributive justice in their social programs, then perhaps some features of Canada's health care system are worth preserving. Sustaining Canada as a just and tolerant democracy is in our view the real sustainability challenge we face together. Thus, as the caretakers of our health care system go about the important and necessary task of modernizing it, we caution them to "First do no harm."

We would like to thank the Atkinson Foundation, its executive director, and trustees for providing most valuable financial support for the entire project. The Atkinson Foundation is also not responsible for any views or errors in this volume. Cathy Fooks and Tony Doob provided throughtful advice and comments throughout the Dialogue project. Vincy Perri provided expert and gracious support to the project throughout. The Institute for Work and Health gave one of us (Terrence Sullivan) the gift of some precious time to complete the project. Vivek Goel encouraged us from the beginning and provided the project with an electronic and financial home at the University of Toronto in the Department of Health Policy, Management, and Evaluation. Malcolm Lester kindly agreed to produce and publish the book in its original edition and gave design and editorial direction to the project rooted in his own deep publishing experience. Thanks are also due to Peter Milroy at UBC Press for his able assistance in getting this second edition into circulation.

Declining Public Confidence in Canada's Health Care System

The establishment of Canada's health care system was a great triumph of citizenship, but after four decades the national program is in a fragile state. In the spring of 2001 the Commission on the Future of Medicare, led by former Saskatchewan premier Roy Romanow, was set up to examine proposals for reform. Many voices have joined the debate. In this short book we will take a look at some of the fundamentals of health care in Canada and examine some promising ideas for sensible reform. We will also argue that certain other approaches, although they seem intuitively to be sound, would actually worsen our problems rather than solve them.[1]

There are many imperfections in our system, and one reads about them daily. All of these imperfections require attention. Canadians hear the cries of alarm and the contradictory solutions that are put forward with regularity. Some critics favour radical surgery for the system, while others opt for a program of incremental change. The voices of panic in this cacophony come from both the left and the right of the political spectrum, from think tanks, employers, and consumers, and from the media, whose attention to the issues often has the effect of magnifying concern and conflict. Thirty-seven percent of Canadians report that their health care opinions are based on what they see or read in the media.[2]

What elements of our system are unique and worth holding on to? In our view, three fundamental aspects of the system now in place are essential and must be retained. First and foremost, *medicare is a subsidy and transfer program.* Through taxation, the public portion of health care is funded by a progressive transfer of money from the better-off levels of our society to provide health services for all on the basis of need. It is supposed to do this, and as we will see shortly, it does so very well. Second, *it's simple*. The single-public-payment mechanism keeps administrative and transaction costs to a minimum, eliminates overheads for sales and competition, and provides a national standard of public coverage for (most) medically necessary services. Third, *it controls costs well* because the bargaining power of a single payer determines how much care we will buy and what kind of deals we can make. A strong single payer can cut better deals with workers, suppliers, and professionals. In our view, any serious reform proposals must retain these three basic features.

These three features are the defining positive elements of our system. But our national system turns on a fourth important feature, the federal government's active role in setting national standards. The role of the federal government contributes some rigidity to our system, which makes change difficult. This rigidity is a positive factor—it means we can't leap into dangerous situations quickly by making precipitous changes and it ensures that Canadians have a health system that reflects their values—but it is also a negative factor for those same reasons—even when fast action is needed, the system is very slow to change. National/intergovernmental consensus is good when it can be achieved, but is elusive. In our view, reform proposals that offer alternatives to the three fundamentals noted above need to be assessed very carefully, and should also be evaluated on how they offer to deal with the rigidity of our system. In an era when government spending is in retreat, and in a country where the fear of provincial secession is always around the corner, a major question facing us on the reform agenda is how a strong federal participation in health care can be mobilized to modernize this most valued of Canadian programs.

CITIZENSHIP, SOLIDARITY, AND CANADIAN VALUES

Our prime minister is always quick to point out that we rank at or near the top of the tables on the UN Human Development Index.[3] Our social programs of old age security, unemployment insurance and health insurance, are supported by a citizenry who have historically placed a high value on a reciprocal responsibility for each other. This reciprocity is embedded in the Canadian Constitution through provisions regarding the equalization of public services from province to province. These provisions ensure the transfer of tax funds from the wealthiest provinces to the poorer ones so that the poorer ones can provide for comparable levels of public service, including health care, with comparable levels of taxation. While the U.S. value system respects, above all, the freedom not to be interfered with, the Canadian Constitution provides for a rich range of rights and freedoms, subject only to such reasonable limits prescribed by law as can be demonstrably justified in a free and democratic society. This uniquely Canadian balance is a much admired constitutional model. We balance the freedom of non-interference with the freedom to choose governments that will act in ways that legitimately constrain individual choice for the public good. Health care is one such area, where, literally in order to save each other's lives, we have constrained (but not prohibited) Canadians' freedom to buy their way to the front of the line. A free choice to buy something you can't afford is no freedom at all.[4]

Free choice for a consumer (who may feel that if he can afford to buy a place at the front of the line, he should be "free" to do so, notwithstanding the lack of any such freedom for others who cannot buy expensive health services) is quite different from free choice for a citizen: universal access to health care, regardless of income, financed through progressive taxation is also a way of expressing freedom and extends that freedom to all citizens.

Work from Manitoba by Cam Mustard and colleagues, shown in Figure 1–1, illustrates simply the subsidy and transfer dimension of public health care in Canada.[5] It shows the progressive pattern of taxation and health care benefits (as health care $ spent for those in each income decile) across the 10 income deciles or tenths of the population in Manitoba. Those in the highest income brackets (decile 10), on average, pay the most taxes and consume the least health care dollars (owing to their superior health). Those in decile 1 (the poorest), where there is the greatest disease burden, derive the greatest benefit in terms of cash equivalents of spending in the health care system. This transfer of benefits based on health *need* is a distinguishing feature of the Canadian health care system. To those who say, "let the wealthy pay for prompt, high-quality care if

they can afford it," we say, "they are paying for it!" They are paying
their own way and also some of the way for the poor, by contribut-
ing in a progressive fashion proportionate to their income. Our
health care system is one very important way in which Canada redis-
tributes the burden of financing health care and health benefits to
its citizens. And, in fact, there is very compelling recent research
suggesting that the way we pool taxes to subsidize health services to
poorer Canadians results in higher overall levels of health in
Canada as compared to the United States.[6]

The argument to allow more choice through "private" spending
often blurs a private consumer argument (we should be allowed to
choose to pay for the health care we want) with a citizenship and
public goods argument (the best health care should be available to
all, not just those who can afford to pay). We all want first-class
health care for our families. In a two-tiered payment system, those
in the private tier opt out of the public plan to buy their way to the

FIGURE 1-1

Incidence of Taxation and Public Health Care Consumption by Economic Family Income Decile, Manitoba 1994

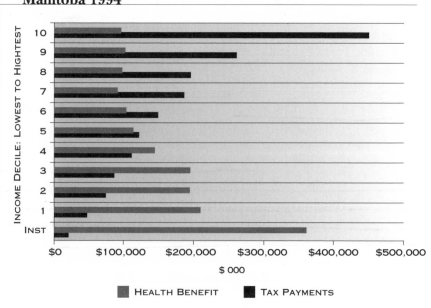

front of the line and those less fortunate wait longer and do not have "choice." This leaves the public tier in a permanent "second class" category. Income and the burden of disease are strongly linked in Canada, as in all countries. Poorer people have poorer health for reasons that have little to do with medical care and only something to with lifestyle. The poor are not less healthy because they are less worthy. Rather, a range of complex factors interacts to produce lower health status among the poor.[7]

Virtually all wealthy nations (the U.S. excluded) ensure some reasonable level of health service for their total population. Canada, however, does not encourage its citizens to buy their way to the front of the line. It is important to note that there is no legal bar to doing this in Canada, although there is a financial penalty to provinces that allow it. Under the law, all citizens in Canada, regardless of income, are entitled to the same quality, timeliness, and level of medically required service, based on their health care needs and not their ability to pay.

While these are worthy Canadian values, we do have serious problems delivering on the promise of one standard of quality. Recently released information from the Canadian Institute for Health Information, for example, shows a threefold variation across regions in Canada in the likelihood of surviving the first thirty days after a heart attack, even with differences in age and income taken into account.[8] Some of this variation in survival may well be explained by factors other than quality of care, but in our view, the reality of that quality and the public's perception of it are equally important: if public support for universal health care begins to erode because of a mistaken belief that it cannot deliver high-quality health services, the future of Canada's health system is in peril.

PUBLIC OPINION SURVEYS IN CANADA

Although a source of national pride and a symbol of Canadian values, the health care system has aroused increasing public concern in the past decade. The public anxiety focuses on issues such as financial sustainability, waiting lists, hospital restructuring and rising private costs. Angus Reid Group[9] found that only 25 percent of Canadians in 2000 rated the health care system and the quality of its

5

services as excellent or very good, compared with 61 percent in 1991.

A slim majority (52 percent) of Canadians give the Canada Health Act a barely passing grade for living up to its principles, and a bigger majority believe that it is time to change the act. The public is no longer entirely sure of the ability of governments to manage social programs.[10] But they are still committed to the five principles on which the system is based: universality, comprehensiveness, accessibility, portability and public administration. On only the last principle was our health system given a failing grade. This is perhaps not surprising, given the decline in deference to public officials in the health sector associated with the Krever Inquiry—the scandal in the Canadian blood system—and the recent deaths in Ontario associated with E. coli in the water in Walkerton. The aspects of health care that concern Canadians most are the ability of the system to provide equal access for all and the continued high quality of the system; the actual cost of the system to the country is not seen as a serious problem. Not surprisingly, therefore, a majority of Canadians still reject the proposition that people who can afford to should be allowed to pay extra to get quicker access to services.[11]

Canadians also express their concern by their ranking of priority issues that governments should deal with. Pollsters, in questioning the public about the setting of priorities by the federal government[12] found that by an overwhelming majority (93 percent) Canadians believe that the federal government should make health care a high priority. Unemployment came in at 77 percent, the national debt at 74 percent, and levels of taxation at 72 percent, indicating that these issues are also given a high priority. But to Canadians, health care reform is urgent.

However, the public respond differently to questions about the health care system depending on whether they have recently had direct experience with it. Even as public concerns grow, Canadians who have had recent direct experience with the health care system are largely quite satisfied with it. The Angus Reid polls show that Canadians who were recently admitted to a hospital, or had a family member admitted for at least one night, say they were satisfied with their stay.[13] Other surveys show that despite the fact that a majority say the system is in crisis and quality has declined, 61 percent believe they will get the care they need if they have a serious medical problem.[14] This same survey found that, overall, patients in Ontario were very satisfied with their inpatient experience.

Some of this growing public concern dates from the 1990s, when both federal and provincial governments cut program costs to reduce the debt and deficit, and, in some provinces, to cut taxes. Cost constraints have also forced provinces to look at smarter ways of delivering services. As a result most provinces have cut hospital budgets and closed down hospitals. Although there has been considerable alarm among the public about these measures, preliminary evidence from some of the provinces shows there has been no reduction in quality or health outcomes. Studies in rural Saskatchewan, urban Winnipeg, and recently, British Columbia have shown that following hospital closures and cutbacks there was no deterioration in the quality of care or the health of the population served (as measured by death rates, hospital readmissions, subsequent emergency room visits, and self-reported levels of health). If anything, the Saskatchewan data suggest that *improved* patient outcomes may be achieved by concentrating larger volumes of specialty care in a smaller number of facilities. The public was alarmed by bed closures, but access to hospital care was shown to be unaffected—the percentage of Manitobans admitted to hospital before and after the closures was unchanged.[15] Despite this, these communities tended to report being dissatisfied with the cuts.

The Ontario Hospital Association's report card of Ontario hospitals also showed that despite the decline in provincial revenues, hospitals were able to increase their efficiency and the resources allocated to patient care. For example, the proportion of total inpatient nursing time spent on nursing care increased over the two years studied; similarly, the proportions of total staff hours spent on patient care increased.[16]

POLLS ACROSS NATIONS

High-quality international surveys[17] of citizens in different countries in recent years provide some interesting insight on how Canada is faring compared to its Commonwealth cousins and the U.S.A. Health reform pressures are being felt in all advanced economies.

Citizens in a number of countries are expressing concern about their health care systems; in fact, concern is growing in all of the countries surveyed. In every case, the nature of the concern reflects the way the system is organized. A survey of Australia, Canada, New Zealand, the United Kingdom, and the United States showed that in each country a majority was not content with their health care system. At one extreme, the U.S. has a strong reliance on private health insurance and a lack of universal coverage. In Britain, at the other extreme, patients generally have access to a broad range of publicly funded medical services and private insurance plays a minor role. Although Canada, like Britain, has universal publicly funded health care, its benefit package is both more expensive than and not as comprehensive as Britain's, leaving a larger role for private insurance. The public health system in Australia and New Zealand are relying more and more on user fees for services included in the public plan and on private insurance as a supplement to public benefits.

Canada and Australia have both experienced a substantial drop in public confidence in their systems over the last decade. However, people in Australia, New Zealand, and the U.S. were more likely than the British or the Canadians to believe that their system required overall change. Americans were more worried about personal affordability of care; Australians and New Zealanders found waiting times and queues to be the biggest problem; the British saw inadequate government funding as the issue; and Canadians were worried not only about government funding but also about government management of the health care system. People in the U.S. and New Zealand were the most likely to report that they had problems paying medical bills and did not always fill prescriptions because the cost was too high. Not surprisingly, these countries have the highest proportion of health spending paid out of pocket: people with lower incomes simply do without medical services if they cannot afford them.

Recent international survey work[18] suggests that the four countries (of the five surveyed) that have universal coverage and also charge user fees and allow a substantial role for private insurance experience the most inequities in care. Figure 1–2 shows the percent of respondents in the four countries with universal coverage

F I G U R E   1 - 2

Percent of Respondents Who Have Private Insurance in Countries with Universal Coverage

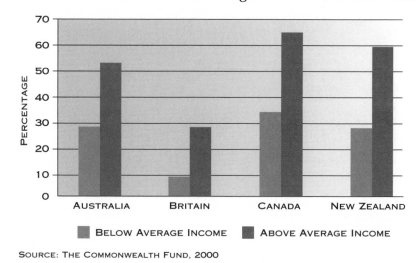

SOURCE: THE COMMONWEALTH FUND, 2000

who have private insurance. Although this private insurance in Canada is supplementary to public health coverage, it gives us a picture of who would have choice in a more privatized insurance market. Private supplemental coverage was widespread among adults with above-average incomes. In the U.S. (not shown) adults with above-average incomes are twice as likely as those with below-average incomes to have private health insurance (84 percent versus 42 percent). People with above-average incomes in the universal coverage countries are able to use private insurance to cover benefits not included in the public plan and (with the exception of Canada) are able to decrease waiting time and gain quicker access to specialists.

The same survey looked at *perceived* access to care. Respondents of below- and above-average income in the five countries are shown in Figure 1–3. Analysis showed a difference in people's perception of access to care between lower- and higher-income groups in Australia, New Zealand, and the U.S. In Canada and Britain, there were no significant differences in perceived access between income groups.

Interestingly enough, in rating whether their country's health

FIGURE 1-3

Percent of Respondents of Below- and Above-Average Income Who Say It Is Difficult to Get Care

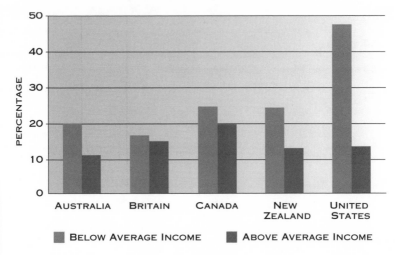

SOURCE: THE COMMONWEALTH FUND, 2000

FIGURE 1-4

Percent of Respondents Who Believe the Health System Needs to Be Completely Rebuilt

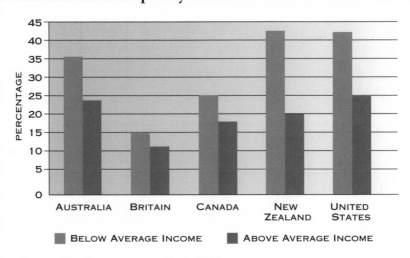

SOURCE: THE COMMONWEALTH FUND, 2000

care system needed complete overhaul, there were different response patterns, as shown in Figure 1–4. Although these recent surveys show that one-fifth of people in Australia, Canada, and the U.S. and only one-tenth of New Zealanders think their system works well and needs only minor changes, these figures hide sharply divided opinions among income groups in Australia, New Zealand, and the U.S., where citizens also report more unequal care experience. The authors of the survey conclude that reliance on market competition—based on direct charges to patients for some services and a major role for private health insurance—appears to incur social costs, driving a wedge in social solidarity.

The mix of public and private financing for health care varies considerably across these five countries, as Figure 1–5 shows. Moreover, health care consumes a lower proportion of gross domestic product (GDP) in countries where public spending is dominant than in countries where multi-payer private spending is permitted.[19]

That public funding makes a difference is supported even by data from the U.S., where there is the heaviest reliance on private spending. In a survey of the elderly, who have nearly universal

FIGURE 1–5

Percent of GDP Spent on Health Care from Public and Private Sources, 1997

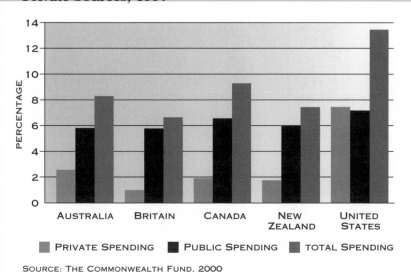

SOURCE: THE COMMONWEALTH FUND, 2000

health insurance coverage through the U.S. Medicare program, response rates to access to care, satisfaction with care, and financial and health-related concerns were similar to those of the elderly in Australia, New Zealand, the U.K., and Canada. There was one significant difference, however, in the U.S. response: they were more concerned about the cost of prescription drugs. Prescription drug costs for the elderly are not covered by U.S. Medicare as they are in the other countries, and American seniors pay higher prices for their drugs than do Canadians.

THE U.S.—SECOND LAST AMONG DEVELOPED COUNTRIES

The irony is that while citizen concern in Canada about the quality of the health care system has been rising in the last few years, most independent, evidence-based assessments of its performance indicate continued improvement, both in the total volume of services provided and in the health outcomes associated with such services. The annual report of the Canadian Institute for Health Information indicates that the life expectancy of Canadians is among the highest in the world, second only to Japan and tied with Iceland. On average, we live approximately two years longer than our American neighbours (who rank twenty-fifth in the world for life expectancy).

Why do we constantly compare ourselves to the U.S? Because it is there. We are not only its neighbour and its biggest trading partner, we also enjoy a largely transparent border. Canadians are bombarded by American media, culture, and ideas, and we tend to see the U.S. as bigger and better in all things. However, in health care this is not the case. While twenty-four of the twenty-nine Organization for Economic Co-operation and Development (OECD) countries ensured that at least 99 percent of their citizens had health insurance coverage in 1997, only three—Mexico, Turkey, and the United States—had no universal coverage. In fact, only 33 percent of the population of the U.S. had government-assured health insurance, while in Mexico the figure was 72 percent and in Turkey 66 percent. Germany and the Netherlands do not require their most affluent citizens to buy health insurance, but nearly all of them do and, therefore, these two countries effectively have universal coverage.[20] The differences in our social programs is an expression of the differences in our values.

Although the U.S. provides less publicly financed insurance for their population, their total spending on health care, from both public and private sources, is overwhelmingly higher than that of other countries (as shown earlier in Figure 1–5). The high cost of health care in the U.S. seems to be tolerated on the assumption that better health results from more expensive care. Many believe the high availability of technology in the U.S. must lead to better outcomes. After all, the U.S. is second only to Japan in the number of magnetic resonance imaging (MRI) units and computed tomography (CT) scanners per million population.[21]

Higher spending, however, does not guarantee better outcomes. Life expectancy in the U.S. is below the OECD median. In 1996, the only infant mortality rates higher than the U.S. were in Hungary, Korea, Mexico, Poland, and Turkey. By nearly all available health outcome measures, the U.S. ranked near the bottom of the OECD countries in 1996, and the rate of improvement for most of the indicators has been slower than the OECD median.[22]

A 1998 study,[23] comparing 13 countries, found that the U.S. ranked an average of twelfth for sixteen available health indicators, including low birth weight; neonatal and infant mortality in years of potential life lost; life expectancy at year 1, year 15, year 40, and year 65; and age-adjusted mortality. Other studies report similar findings. Canada ranked third behind Japan and Sweden. These findings were confirmed in the 2000 World Health Organization annual report.[24]

Moreover, not only do Americans compare unfavourably on most health indicators, there is also evidence that an estimated 44,000 to 98,000 Americans die each year due to medical errors.[25] U.S. estimates of the combined effect of errors and adverse effects from iatrogenic causes (complications or illness caused by medical examination or treatment) total 225,000 deaths per year. This means, unbelievable as it may seem, that medical errors constitute the third leading cause of death in the U.S., after deaths from heart disease and cancer.[26] Clearly, higher spending on health care and the availability of the most recent innovations and technology do not necessarily translate into better health.

On almost every health status indicator, Canada ranks higher than the U.S. This does not mean that we should feel complacent in any way. There are problems in our health care system that warrant immediate attention, and the recent rise in public concern is driving political attention. People are unhappy about waiting for specialty care and high-technology procedures, and worried about the growing burden of informal care and pharmaceutical costs associated with a shift in care from hospitals to the community. Transferring the responsibility for those services to the community means that provinces are no longer required to insure them as publicly paid services, according to the funding criteria and sanctions of the Canada Health Act. While most provinces provide some publicly funded community care, these services are discretionary, not comprehensive and not held to a national standard across the country.[27]

INTERNATIONAL TRADE AGREEMENTS

Canada is not unique in having structural problems in its health care system and needing to address them. However, there are also threats to our system from outside of our borders. International trade agreements are designed to make national borders permeable to allow for the expansion of free trade, and most such agreements exempt public health and social programs.[28] Nonetheless, there is growing concern—as was seen on television screens around the world in the demonstrations at the World Trade Organization's talks in Seattle and against the Free Trade Agreement of the Americas. Concerns have been expressed by a broad range of consumer groups, environmentalists, trade unions, and public-health activists that international trade agreements may be avenues for the privatization of education, health, welfare, social housing, and transportation. Powerful multinational corporations in the medical, pharmaceutical, insurance, and service industries are pushing for the right to provide these services on a privatized, commercial basis, hoping to capture and enlarge some of the very significant gross domestic product currently spent on them.[29 30]

Some governments have agreed to deregulate and privatize the funding and delivery of certain public services. They are largely doing this through the commercial contracting out of service delivery (such as hospital care in Alberta and home care in Ontario) and through the privatization of public infrastructure (the Toronto Hospital recently issued a large bond to finance infrastructure renovations) and the de-insurance of some public services. Two legal opinions obtained by concerned groups have advised that Alberta's Bill 11 may open the door for American and Mexican health providers to enter the Canadian system. Once they are in, it may be very hard to get them out: it could be prohibitively expensive for Canadian governments to return to a made-in-Canada health care system.[31] [32] As health care goes to market, policy decisions and accountability for those decisions move from the public sphere of accountable governments to unaccountable, private corporate boardrooms and the binding settlements of international trade panels.

National governments, too, increasingly perceive themselves as accountable not only to their own citizens but also to off-shore companies who can sue them for unfair treatment in international courts.[33] The new consumerism that trumpets individual rights is matched by this growth of uncivic corporate investment and trade rights, that challenge the traditions of public solidarity on which our health care programs are based. So the manner in which we balance the public and the private aspects of our health care system, now and for the future, also has important implications for future outcomes in trade and investment disputes.

THREE VOICES OF CONCERN

The Canadian health care system has faced significant difficulties in the past decade. Real spending on health care *declined* through the 1990s. Following the recession of 1990–91, federal and provincial governments bore down dramatically on health care spending, particularly in the area of hospital services, which resulted in a real drop in health care spending between 1990 and 1997. These moves came in response to pressure from international financial bodies because of the rapid expansion of our debt. In the last couple of years, health care spending has begun to grow again. However, the legacy of the earlier fiscal squeeze on the health care system in

Canada is still significant. Moreover, the downward pressure affected some actors more than others.

Public sentiment is heavily influenced by the thousands of messages arriving from the U.S. media—and from some key Canadian voices as well—on a daily basis, proclaiming the excellence of American health care.[34] With respect to health care, these voices promote discontent and public anxiety. Their motives and interests differ, but the noise they generate has the same effect: it erodes public confidence. In a publicly financed universal social program like Canadian health care, which relies on political consensus, this is one of the more serious of the problems that plague our system.

First among the Canadian voices criticizing the system is that of the providers and professionals, especially organized medicine, but to a lesser extent, nursing as well. The fiscal pressures of the mid-nineties and the consequent decline in real public health care spending during that period of time put enormous pressures on the community of professional providers in Canada. This translated into income pressure on organized medicine and also into real and measurable intensification of the burdens of medical practice, especially in the hospital sector, and a stepped-up pressure to treat patients "sicker and quicker." Many of the budget cuts in hospitals throughout the 1990s were accomplished through reductions in the number and type of nurses practising in those settings. We are now facing nursing shortages as the cohort of current nurses ages without sufficient numbers being trained to replace them. Nurses have also experienced an intensification of their workload arising from a more acutely ill and more complex group of hospital in-patients. While hospitals experience nursing shortages, the differential wage scales between institutional and community settings create even greater pressures on nursing personnel in home care. As a result, providers, especially nurses, do face dramatic pressures and show distinctive patterns of job stress.[35]

Physicians and nurses understandably have expressed grave concerns and worries about conditions in the health care system and they have been at the front of the queue calling for more resources and raising concerns about declining quality. The voices of health care providers are not simply self-interested, although it would be a mistake to believe that self-interest is not part of calls for job security for nurses or income stability for physicians. The Canadian health care system was built on compromises negotiated between government and providers, especially organized medicine. We now need to add nurses to the compromise and accommodate their demands.[36] When the provider community is distressed, patients are the first recipients and multipliers of that distress.

The second voice frequently heard is that of private vendors of technology, insurance, and private health services. These participants naturally call for a stronger role for private payment, private access to capital markets, and private delivery. This is not a criticism of the role of private vendors, but an observation on the obvious: their voices reflect their self-interest. They are promoting private solutions in order to increase their market share. To date we have resisted their exhortations in the area of most medically necessary services. But today, as health care shifts from hospitals to the home, we must weigh medical necessity against social necessity. Sometimes the line blurs between what should be publicly funded and what may be privately funded.

There is now and always has been an important place in Canada for the role of private initiatives. This is especially true now in innovations involving information and medical technology. From hand-held blood-testing devices to imaging machines and gene-splitting science, technological innovations created by private industry offer enormous promise both as life-saving and as labour-saving mechanisms.

Truth be told, we have only just begun to adapt to the *telephone* as a technology to support health service delivery and to organize care on the basis of need. And notwithstanding a range of legitimate privacy concerns, privately owned information systems and technologies not only support institutional and community care, but are also a valuable management resource in modernizing health care delivery, improving access to and quality of care, and effectively reducing and managing wait lists. As indicated earlier, however, there are less noble motives in the health industry for increasing private financing.

The third voice comes from political ideologues of both the right and the left. The right advocates more private money and more "choice." What this means, in practice, is usually the creation of a second tier of health care available only to those able to pay for it. It is often suggested that this would be a way to free up more resources for the public system. The left, for its part, argues that cuts to our system have severely impaired its quality and that our system is underfunded and on the verge of collapse. They argue that unless we pump more money into the system, overall quality (and the security of employment) will deteriorate. Thus right and left appear to agree that the system is not working. This unlikely and unintended coalition of politically incompatible critics is troubling. Although they have different interests and goals, their voices create a chorus that fragments public consensus and weakens our resolve to change what should be changed while preserving the essential principles of the Canadian health care system. A more demanding public, frightened by the declarations of doom, may not be able to see the difference between financial and merely managerial problems.

In all of this, the media have a special role in reporting the complaints of unhappy providers, private vendors, and ideologues. Because the media are attracted by stories of conflict and disagreement, they tend to project a polarized view of any situation they comment on, even when there are many sides to a debate and the difference in evidence among the multiple positions is stark and unequivocal. Despite their inclination to conclude blandly that the truth lies somewhere in between the extreme positions, truth is never found somewhere between sense and nonsense.

This role of the media in the promotion of discontent was highlighted in thoughtful commentaries recently published by Ted Marmor from Yale University in both Canadian and U.S. news publications.[37] He noted that Canadian stories on emergency room problems at the height of the influenza season in February were virtually identical with the U.S. stories, with one major difference: both the Canadian and U.S. stories blamed the Canadian problem on the "frayed fabric" of our health care system, while the problems reported in American hospitals (which were no less dramatic) could not be attributed to such an obvious source and were blamed on situational and episodic factors such as an understandable increase in emergency room visits during the flu season. As Marmor points out, domestic interests in the U.S. often promote these different attributions of the problem. The richest among these groups want, specifically, to attack the Canadian model. A less generous Canadian assessment of the problems in U.S. emergency rooms would be that there is no public accountability or planning for delays or blockages in ERs. It just "happens." The perennial solution offered by throwing money at hospitals for emergency room crowd-ing overlooks some of the preventative (non-hospital) solutions that have been proposed or used successfully elsewhere: population-based flu vaccinations to reduce peak winter ER visits and the reform of physician payment methods to ensure that GPs are avail-able to see patients after hours. The latter would take more than money to put into effect; it calls for a reorganization of physicians' offices and their after-hours practice arrangements,[38] a reorganiza-tion that to date has been hampered by a lack of political will.

The weak economic performance in 2001 has once again prompted fiscal concerns from governments in Canada as public revenues slow or fall. The infusion of almost $20 billion by the fed-eral government in the fall of 2000 muted public worry for a while but there is now increasing talk about the "sustainability" of growth in health spending as a proportion of government spending in Canada. Yet health spending as a percentage of all public spending has grown continuously for four decades. No magic threshold at which sustainability falters has been defined.

But the pollsters say, perception *is* what matters and, at the end of the day, public perceptions are less shaped by evidence than by interests. We need to strengthen the core of evidence while at the same time emphasizing the ways in which a public health care sys-tem is in everybody's interest. Public opinions are formed on the basis of personal experience and on media reports on health issues, which as we noted are often caricatures of reality. The facts must be presented to the public clearly and forcefully, as some of the new Health Report Cards from the Canadian Institute for Health Information are attempting to do. Another approach is to raise other voices.

In this short volume we will revisit the value and the principles of our health financing arrangements in Canada, while acknowl-edging the urgency of some of the pressing changes that need to be made in the organization and management of health services and in the range of services covered.

What Is Public and What Is Private?

FISCAL FEDERALISM

Canada is often described by others as a federation with fairly clear boundaries between the federal and provincial governments.[1] Health care is one of the areas where the provinces have legal authority for organizing and providing services. The federal government cannot legitimately legislate or regulate health care issues (with some narrow exceptions related to aboriginal and public health). It can, however, steer what provinces do through its spending power. Using the major federal instrument of transfer to the provinces, the Canada Health and Social Transfer (CHST) Act, the federal government transfers funding to the provinces for post-secondary education, health care and welfare services. In exchange for this federal money, the provinces must accept certain conditions for health care, and the federal government is able to ensure that the provinces conform to these conditions through the penalty of withholding funds for a breach. This "spending power" is effectively the basis for a national health care standard in Canada.

In addition to this balancing of provincial jurisdiction for health care against federal spending power, Canadians benefit from another unique constitutional feature related to health: under the equalization provisions of the Canadian Constitution, the provinces are obliged to provide "reasonably comparable levels of public service for reasonably comparable levels of taxation." Total spending (from both public and private sources) on health care in Canada in 1999 was just under $3,000 per person; the public portion was just under $2,000 per person. Figure 2–1 shows that the per capita public spending on health care in each province is reasonably similar.

FIGURE 2-1

Overall Spending Per Capita in Each Province Is Quite Similar 1999

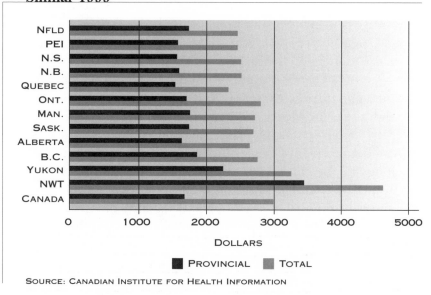

SOURCE: CANADIAN INSTITUTE FOR HEALTH INFORMATION

Given the unequal wealth of the provinces due to variation in the size of their tax bases, the federal government transfers tax money from the "have" provinces (e.g. B.C., Alberta, Ontario) to the "have-not" provinces (e.g., the Atlantic and other provinces) to assist them in providing reasonably comparable levels of public service for reasonably comparable levels of taxation. The mechanism for effecting the transfer is the Equalization Program, second only to the Canada Health and Social Transfer in the amount of public money it handles. As a result, the have-not provinces are doubly dependent; they must look not only to the federal government but also to the "have" provinces for health care financing.

The federal spending through the CHST comes as a mixture of cash transfers to the provinces and "tax points" from income tax. With respect to the "tax points" portion, the federal government agreed to reduce its tax rate, thereby allowing the provincial governments to increase theirs without affecting the total taxes that the taxpayer must pay. Federal payments to the provinces for health care have indeed dropped—from roughly 40 percent of all public spending on health care in the mid-1970s to less than a third in the mid-1990s.

THE CANADA HEALTH ACT

The story of the evolution of the health care system in Canada has been well told by others, but it's worth noting that it did start as an innovative provincial program that then became national through federal spending support. The federal involvement initially underwrote the training of doctors, the building of hospitals, and the early provision of doctors' care and hospitalization insurance in Canada. Hospital and physicians' services remain the core services covered through the principles of the Canada Health Act (CHA). The CHA basically requires that in order to receive federal transfers, the provinces must meet five specific program criteria. It is also worth restating that the only effective authority the federal government has to promote a national program is the power to add or withhold spending, conditional on the provinces' meeting the CHA criteria.

The first CHA criterion is *public administration*: health insurance be administered and operated on a not-for-profit basis by a public authority appointed or designated by the government or the province.[2] The second criterion is *comprehensiveness*: the health care plan of a province must insure *all* medically necessary health services provided by hospitals, medical practitioners and, where the law permits, additional services rendered by other health care practitioners. (This question of what is covered has become the most challenging problem in our current system as insured care increasingly moves outside hospitals and into the community, where it no longer is covered by the conditions of the CHA). The third criterion is *universality*: the health care insurance plan of a province must cover 100 percent of the insured people in the population on uniform terms and conditions. The fourth criterion is *portability*: some provision must be made to cover, on a relatively uniform basis, citizens travelling from one province to another and outside the country, allowing for interprovincial and international recovery of costs. The last criterion is *accessibility*: the plan must provide insured services on uniform terms and conditions that do not impede or preclude reasonable access to the services through any form of private charges; and the province must provide "reasonable" compensation for insured services rendered by medical practitioners and pay hospitals for the cost of insured health services.

Under the CHA, mention is made of extended health services including nursing homes, intermediate care, adult residential care, home care services and ambulatory care services. Although some funds were provided for these health services, no strings are attached to this money and extended health services do not have to meet the five criteria. The consequence is that while levels of overall spending by province in Canada are, relatively, comparable, the hidden reality is that there is a threefold variation in public spending support across the provinces in extended health services like home care and pharmaceuticals.

This is the real challenge in the reform of the Canadian health care system. The legacy of health insurance in Canada, i.e. insurance for doctors' care and hospitals, is not really keeping pace with the most significant change that is occurring: the transfer of services to the community. This is so because the federal government does not require that extended community services, home care, long-term care, and pharmaceuticals be provided under the same terms and conditions as physician's and hospital services, notwithstanding the fact that many pharmaceuticals would be considered medically necessary and some acute care services are now provided in the home. In short, the federal financing mechanism (conditional funding transfers) that we have in this country is very effective for medical and hospital care and is very successful at maintaining and delivering the three key elements of our system, as noted in Chapter 1 (public subsidy, simplicity, and cost control). But we have no effective means of controlling costs or establishing national standards for pharmaceuticals, or for care provided in the home and the community. There were no conditions placed on the large amount of new CHST money that the federal government transferred to the provinces as a result of the fall 2000 First Ministers' meeting. This apparent political reluctance to reshape what is required by the federal government is our single biggest "rigidity challenge."

HEALTH SPENDING IN CANADA

Although federal spending has a very important steering effect on health care in Canada, it represents a minority of spending from province to province. While we're spending about $3,000 per per-

F I G U R E   2 - 2

Federal Health Transfers in 1992 Dollars Per Capita

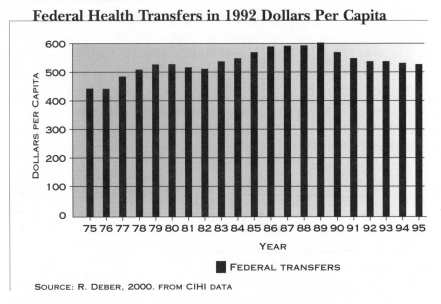

SOURCE: R. DEBER, 2000. FROM CIHI DATA

son in Canada (Figure 2–1), Figure 2–2 shows the federal transfers to the provinces at just over $500 per capita for the last few years (using 1992 dollars—actual dollars have risen, but 1992 dollars allow for real increases by adjusting for inflation). Federal payments have dropped from about 40 percent of all public spending in health care in the 1970s to less than a third in the 1990s.

Taking into account the fact that the Canadian population has been growing at the same time, it is more meaningful to look at the change in health spending per person (per capita) over the years to get a clearer picture of whether we are, on average, spending more or less for each Canadian over time. Figure 2–3 shows precisely this, and from it we can see the emergence of a slightly different trend in public and private spending from that indicated in Figure 2–2. Figure 2–3 shows health spending per capita from 1975 to 1997 separated into private, provincial (which includes federal transfers), and other public. While private spending continued to grow, what is more significant is the modest decline in real provincial spending in the early 1990s. This is the first such decline in health spending in Canadian history. It was the predictable consequence of the massive fiscal pressure arising from debt and the recession of the early

FIGURE 2 - 3

Canadian Health Spending in 1992 Dollars Per Capita 1975 to 1997

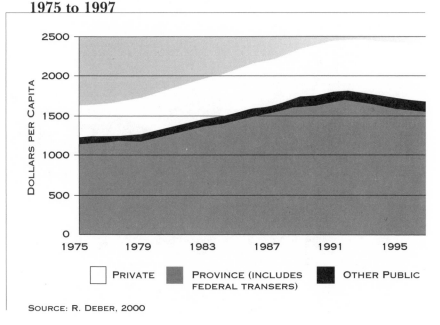

SOURCE: R. DEBER, 2000

1990s. This fiscal pressure, as we have stated, drove the reduction of federal transfers to the provinces in the mid-1990s.

The predictable consequences of this reduction in federal transfer payments, as discussed in Chapter 1, included a massive downward pressure on hospital and medical services in particular, but the squeeze was also felt across all of the publicly financed health care sector. At the same time, the growth of privately financed services has been continuous. The result of these changes has been a shift in the balance between public and private financing of health care.

Figure 2–4 shows the total spending in health care in Canada broken down into provincial (which includes the federal transfers), private, and other public (which includes Workers' Compensation, municipal spending, and federal spending on native reserves and for veterans). Spending in Canada in 2001 will be in the range of $100 billion a year, making health care a colossal industry sector.

FIGURE 2-4

Canadian Health Spending in $ Millions 1975 to 1999

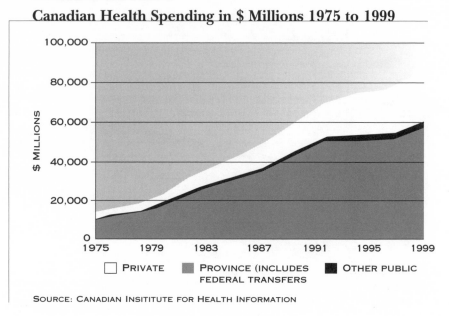

SOURCE: CANADIAN INSITITUTE FOR HEALTH INFORMATION

INTERNATIONAL COMPARISONS

How does health spending in Canada compare with other countries? Do we spend more on health care in total than other countries?

Figure 2–5 shows total health spending in Canada as a percentage of gross domestic product (GDP), that is, the proportion of our national wealth that is spent on health care, comparing Canada to the U.S., the U.K., and a 22-country average of OECD nations. What's worth noting is that Canada is marginally above the 22-country average and well above the U.K., but well below the U.S. spending totals. The U.S. is the odd-man-out in the international spending community by a country mile, but as we showed in Chapter 1, it does not get a proportionate result in better health outcomes for its higher amount of spending.

There are three things to note from Figure 2–5. First, Canada and the U.S. spent about the same proportion of GDP on health care until the early 1970s, when Canada introduced universal health insurance. The increasing difference in spending between Canada

FIGURE 2-5

Total Health Spending as a Percentage of GDP

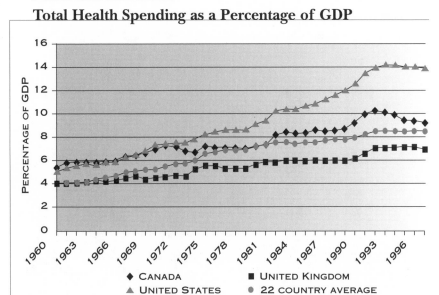

SOURCE: R. DEBER, 2000. FROM ORGANIZATION FOR ECONOMIC COOPERATION AND DEVELOPMENT (OECD) DATA

and the U.S. since that time in part has to do with the greater cost control and simplicity arising from the single-payer approach to health insurance. The second thing to note in Figure 2–5 is that the modest downturn in the early 1990s in health spending as a proportion of GDP in Canada is consistent with the actual reductions in cash and per capita spending. The third point to notice is that Canada nevertheless spends somewhat more than the OECD 22-country average.

PUBLIC VERSUS PRIVATE COVERAGE

In the federal election in the fall of 2000, there was much loose talk about public and private issues in health care. To establish the facts in the matter, let's now consider what health care is publicly financed and what is paid for privately. Remember that through the mixture of largely provincial and some federal dollars, Canada manages to finance a "reasonably comprehensive" range of services. You will note from Figure 2–6 that the actual 1998 public share of spending is quite significant for doctors (98.7 percent), hospitals (91.1

FIGURE 2 - 6

Public and Private Shares of Total Health Expenditure by Use of Funds, Current Dollars, Canada, 1998

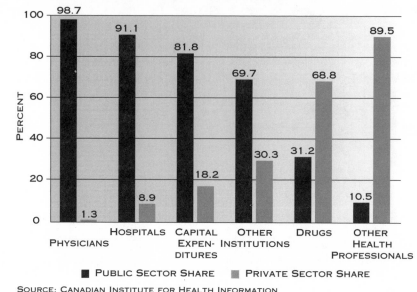

SOURCE: CANADIAN INSTITUTE FOR HEALTH INFORMATION

percent), capital expenditures (81.8 percent), and other institutions (69.7 percent), but is a minority of spending for drugs (31.2 percent) and other health professionals (10.5 percent). When Canada first introduced universal health insurance, medical and hospital care were the high-cost items. As a result, public financing protected Canadians from the catastrophic costs associated with these services. However, the site and nature of care has shifted from the hospital to the home where more complex care can be provided through improved but expensive technology and pharmaceuticals. However, the legacy of our early commitments to health care (public payment for medical and hospital care) has not changed to meet this new reality. In short, the continued emphasis on public payment for medical and hospital care no longer offers the same comprehensive protection for Canadians from financial risk as it did in the past.

When we talk about the problems with our health care system, we talk about it as a uni-dimensional beast. But in fact we need to separate out the different dimensions of this policy. We can't have a useful discussion about problems in health care or the role of government unless we separate financing—the payment—from purchasing and from the provision of care. Policy analysts often refer to the three dimensions as *financing* (who pays for what services for whom); *allocation* (what mechanisms does the payer use to purchase service from the deliverer); and *delivery* (who provides the services). In simple terms, we can separate the elements of a health care system into these three dimensions that lie along a public-private continuum and can vary greatly from country to country.

➤ **Financing** can vary along a continuum from public to private resources.

➤ **Allocation** or purchase of services can be done through direct transfers from government or through more quasi-market mechanisms, such as competitive contracting-out by public purchasing authorities or by competitive purchasing within a for-profit health management organization (HMO), as is frequently the case in the U.S. It can vary from complete government control to a completely free market.

➤ **Delivery** of services can be provided by the public, by not-for-profit bodies, by a regulated for-profit sector, or by unregulated for-profit providers.

By choosing different points along the continuum for each dimension, countries have developed different health care systems. Table 2–1 gives examples of how these dimensions are handled in Canada's health care arrangements.

To correctly diagnose the problems in health care systems and come up with effective solutions, we must be clear about which of these three dimensions we are focusing on. For example, the problem of waiting lists may have to do with not enough money (financing), how we pay hospitals and providers (allocation), or inadequate information and management systems (delivery). If the problem is inadequate management systems, throwing more money at the delivery system without introducing better management on information systems is a waste and will not solve our problems.

This schema simplifies the elaborate flow of funds (shown in Figure 2–7) in the Canadian health care system. This diagram

TABLE 2 – 1

Different Versions of Public and Private in Health Care

	FINANCE	ALLOCATION	DELIVERY
PUBLIC	Tax Pooling for Health Ministry	Provincial or Federal $ to Hospitals vs. Community Care vs. Education and Training	Municipal Public Health Services
PRIVATE NOT-FOR-PROFIT	Charities, Foundations, and some Health Research Agencies	Regional Health Authorities to Hospitals vs. Home Care vs. Primary Care	Public Hospitals Community Health Centres
FOR-PROFIT	Private Insurance and Payroll Group Health Benefits	Managed Care Corporations (in the U.S.)	Cosmetic Surgery Clinics Nursing Homes Private Labs

illustrates the complexities of diagnosing the source of problems and developing meaningful solutions.

About 70 percent of all health care payment is public, which means that about 30 percent of health services purchased in Canada come out of private insurance or out of people's pockets. The public portion of *financing* comes from general revenue and taxation and a very small amount of money comes from payroll premiums levied by some provincial governments.

Allocation decisions as to how money is distributed and how services are *purchased* are largely provincial responsibilities that are, outside of Ontario, carried out by regional authorities. Most provinces in Canada now have some form of regional health authority that plays a role in the allocation of money and the purchase of services. The funder may directly transfer the money to the hospitals and providers (as the government in Ontario does) or to regional authorities (in other provinces) that, in turn, transfer funds to hospitals. Or the purchaser/funder may hold competitions among

FIGURE 2-7

Health Care Financing Flows in Canada

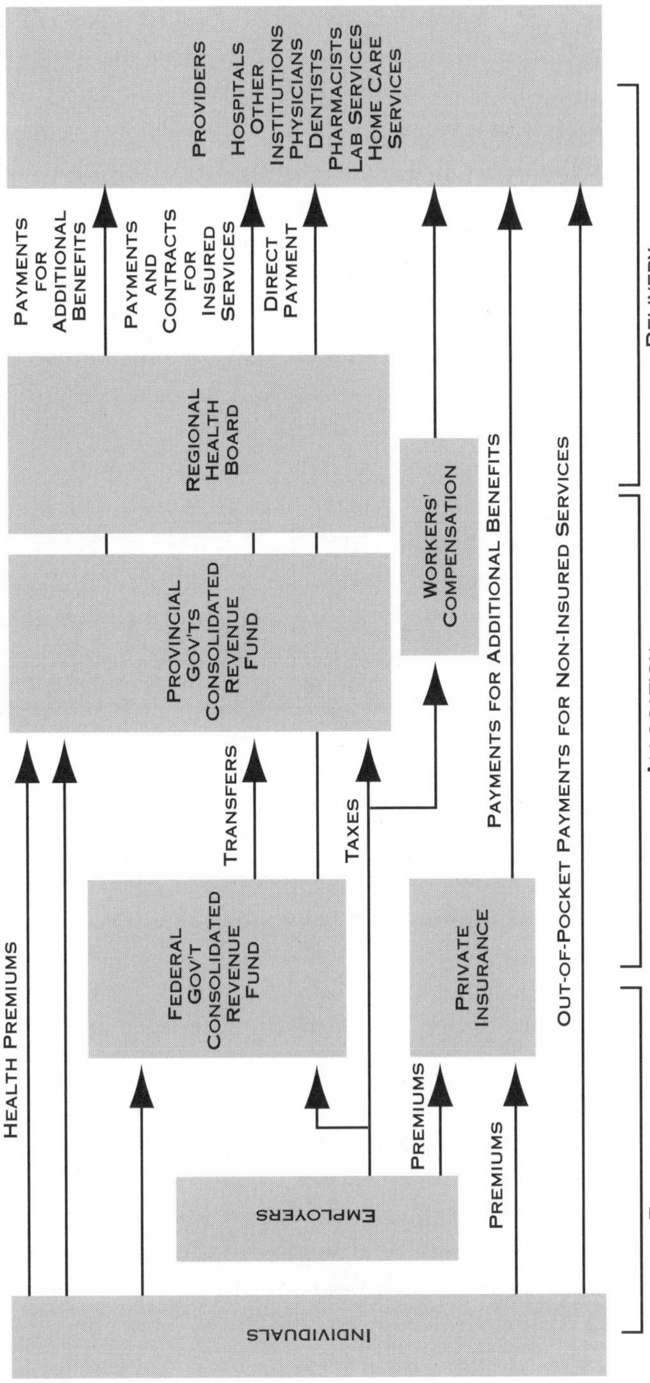

for-profit and not-for-profit providers for contracts to deliver services, as the Community Care Access Centres do in Ontario for home care and as many jurisdictions do for lab services.

At the level of delivery, Canada has a largely private delivery system. Most hospitals are private not-for-profit corporations operating under provincial legislation. Likewise, physicians and most laboratory services operate within a "private realm." In a number of provinces physicians can incorporate as private businesses. So Canada has a national health care system where about 70 percent of the financing comes from general taxation but almost all of the delivery is private. We have always had, in this sense, a unique "public-private" partnership.

The recent controversy in Alberta about "private" hospitals stemmed largely from the concern over for-profit *delivery* of hospital care. In our view, the immediate problem is the creeping growth of supplementary fees (private financing) and the longer-term issue of the opening of our borders to American for-profit health care corporations. In the Alberta proposal, patients can receive publicly funded care in for-profit hospitals, i.e. publicly paid services in a facility that exists to make a profit. One of the easiest ways to make a profit is to introduce add-ons or deluxe services for a supplementary fee premium—a move that opens the door to a second "tier" of health care for those who can afford it. The expansion of Canadian for-profit providers may allow American corporations to sue for equal treatment, claiming that it is their right under international trade agreements to set up in Canada. Once in Canada, they will drive the wedge between public and private even deeper, creating additional pressure to privatize both the financing and the delivery of health care.

SO, WHAT ABOUT CONSUMER "CHOICE"?

Much of the current debate turns on the extent to which, in the era of e-health—Internet health information and services—and consumer sovereignty, consumers should be able to choose their doctors, and to buy their way to the front of the line for private health care. In fact, patients in Canada have extraordinary choice. They can choose any physician or hospital they wish without impediment or barrier and without incurring any additional charges. There is no central "Soviet-style" mechanism that limits patient choice in terms of where they may go. What *is* limited is the right of wealthy people to buy their way to the front of the line, even when poorer people's health problems are more severe (as on an average they tend to be).

This is in stark contrast to the U.S. where there is a very regressive relationship between financing and health care use.[3] That is, the poor pay more out-of-pocket and derive less benefit from the services they buy than the very wealthy. We are speaking here of the poor who can afford to get health care at all, since at the last count approximately 43 million people in the U.S. had no health insurance, and an additional unascertainable but certainly large number are underinsured. As we stated earlier, the Canadian system covers virtually all hospital and medical costs. These health costs can be quite catastrophic and variable if they are borne by the individual. In the U.S. these are the sectors that generate very large personal bills that force numbers of Americans into bankruptcy. What is more, in the U.S., fewer lower-income people are getting employer-sponsored coverage.[4]

The freedom in the U.S. to buy one's way to the front of the line through a set of competing insurance arrangements is also a recipe for escalating costs, and it creates a system that Marcia Angell, the former editor of the *New England Journal of Medicine,* called "the most expensive and the most inadequate system in the developed world." Far from being the Mecca of personal choice, average Americans do not have much discretion over who their physician or provider is, since they are typically committed to a particular HMO or preferred provider network as a function of their payroll benefits. Nor are doctors and other service providers able to exercise levels of discretion or professional autonomy comparable to those of Canadian doctors and providers, since they are subject to more careful investigation, with complex requirements for prior approval of health insurance benefits, concurrent care review, and retrospective audits. As a result, decisions about treatment by American physicians are subject to much more bureaucratic inquisition and control. These differences in how doctors are paid and scrutinized in Canada and the U.S. have been likened to fences versus reins on the providers.[5] Canada tends to constrain providers through a set of overall budget caps and overall publicly bargained negotiations with physicians' associations (fences), whereas Americans tend to micro-manage at the level of individual physicians and individual competitive organizations (reins). As a result, while American providers, especially physicians, may make more income, they have far less independence in their professional decisions than Canadian doctors.

As stated earlier, the Canadian health care system is one in which about 70 percent of the spending comes from public sources, largely through general taxation and a small proportion through payroll deductions in some provinces. This public spending is steered in part by the conditions imposed through the federal government and the CHA, which, in addition to imposing some cost constraints, also acts as a political and moral force compelling the provinces to provide the same health care to all. The Canadian system is solidly within the average of and marginally above most of our European comparators in terms of the amount of money spent on health care. Although Canadians may have a European model of universal insurance, they have a very North American delivery model with a largely private and largely (but not exclusively) not-for-profit delivery system. Despite rhetoric to the contrary, the Canadian public and its health care providers have much more choice and autonomy in our health care system than their counterparts in the market-driven U.S. system.[6]

The big challenge in Canada remains how to ensure the continued success of our methods of financing medically necessary services, and, at the same time, to adjust what provinces are compelled to cover, expanding the historical base of hospital and doctors' services to a modern one that includes services such as home care and pharmaceuticals. Despite the rigidities of our transfer arrangements, provinces must somehow be compelled to pay for or allocate money to new services that are not currently covered by the CHA. While nothing in the CHA currently *prevents* any province from paying for a more comprehensive range of health care services, neither does anything in our current arrangements *compel* them to do so (and they are not likely to do so voluntarily). The CHA only compels the funding of physician and hospital services, making those the only areas in which we have national standards. The federal government has historically played an important role, but it is not clear today that it has the conviction to institute serious reform. Unless the federal government is willing to present the provinces with new conditions for additional money (a politically touchy proposition), disparities between the provinces will grow in the crucial areas of home care, pharmaceutical coverage, and other services not included in current conditions for cost sharing. In the fall of 2000 neither the federal (nor the provincial) governments showed any interest in establishing new conditions. The federal government simply gave the provinces a pile of new money, with a nod to some renewal, without trying to extend a base of coverage for home care to all Canadians.

The federal government faces a difficult trade-off: if it asserts its spending power, it alienates Quebec and some other provinces (which object to *any* conditional federal transfers). At the end of the day the government of Canada will either accommodate these provinces or establish national standards. In fact, the federal government already has a political mechanism to do both, by allowing for what is called "asymmetry," as it has done in the case of the Quebec pension plan. According to this formula, as long as the federal government is satisfied that Quebec's solution meets the national objective, it can release funds. However, in recent years it has backed away from imposing any conditions on transfers, a situation that has left us adrift in the very areas that urgently require some national standard (home care, pharmaceutical care). Following the recommendations of the National Forum on Health, the federal government has made a commitment to reform in these areas, but so far has not delivered.[7]

Memes and Myths

A meme[1] is an idea that self-replicates and makes its way into common culture, regardless of its merits. A kind of cultural DNA or virus, memes are contagious information patterns that replicate by parasitically infecting human minds and altering their behaviour, causing them to propagate the pattern. The term was coined by analogy with "gene." Individual slogans, catchphrases, melodies, icons, inventions, and fashions are typical memes. Ironically, unlike genes, the fitness of the meme is not necessarily related to the fitness that it confers on human beings who hold and perpetuate them. The "smoking is cool" meme, for example, may do very well in selling cigarettes while killing off its hosts at a great rate. The notion that "more private money and more competitive insurance will fix our problem of cost escalation" is a meme in our view: one that is continuously served up as a remedy for health reform in our country.[2]

There is a strong consensus among knowledgeable international analysts that the serious problems in Canada's health care system relate not to financing but to allocation and delivery: how we purchase services and get them to people who need them. Nevertheless, some of the concern currently stems from myths about our single-public-payer structure and false hopes associated with proposals for increased private finance.

After all, if the problem is that costs are skyrocketing and waiting lists are growing because of a lack of funding, and if people are willing to pay privately for health care, why *not* allow some private financing to relieve the pressure on our strained health care system? It seems to make intuitive sense. This chapter addresses some of these issues and clarifies some of the assumptions underlying them.

HEALTH CARE AS HAMBURGERS

People who advocate private financing of health care usually do so on the premise that it is like any other good or service you can buy on the market. Let us examine this supposition through examples.

There once was a very interesting debate between two physicians: one an aspiring dean of medicine and the other a young primary-care physician/epidemiologist, about whether health care should or should not be sold like hamburgers. It is a common debate and, frankly, a little silly. Consider the following examples.[3]

1. You are hungry and homeless and you go to a McDonald's and order a meal. You don't have enough money to pay. Should they give you the food?
2. You have just won the option to buy a brand new Mercedes for $500. The only catch is that you have to pick it up within the next three months. Do you accept?

Most people would agree with the predictable market outcome that the fast-food outlet doesn't have to feed you. Most people also would be delighted to have the option to buy a car for $500 no matter when they can get it. Now consider two similar scenarios in the health sector.

1A. You come to emergency with chest pain from a heart attack and you don't have enough money to pay for admission. Should you be treated?
2A. A healthy person has just won the option of a lung transplant in the hospital of his/her choice for $500. The only catch is that the transplant must be taken in the next three months. Does he/she accept?

Suddenly the normal economic laws of supply and demand in a free marketplace do not seem to make sense. Most people would agree that your heart attack should be treated since you are in danger of dying, and that as a society we would be willing to cover your costs if you cannot. This means that you shouldn't be allowed to be priced out of the market for a service that might save your life. The second scenario, of the offer of the reduced-price transplant, highlights the fact that health care is driven not by desire or demand but by need. No one would subject themselves to a surgical procedure unless it was necessary (with the possible exception of discretionary procedures like cosmetic surgery and corrective lens surgery) just because it was cheap.

In a free country, so the argument goes, people should be free to spend their money as they see fit. However, our example illustrates a couple of the important differences between health care and ordinary market goods and services. And, there is, in addition, the perverse incentive (conflict of interest) that may lead providers to recommend unnecessary care because that is how they make a living. Patients do not usually have the ability or resources to inform themselves sufficiently to make decisions about "buying" care. Even for an informed consumer the warning in *caveat emptor* (buyer beware) would be difficult to heed in an open market for health care. Indeed, this is why health care operates most effectively and safely in a very carefully regulated environment. This means no one is free to check him- or herself into hospital for surgery, chemotherapy, or radiation without the express consent and permission of a licensed and regulated physician. Allowing people to buy the care they *want* confuses people's real desires with fundamental human need, and naively blurs the massive asymmetry of knowledge between patients and providers.

For these reasons, although health care is often referred to as a public good, it is one that many people feel cannot and should not be bought and sold according to the laws of the market. Indeed, in economic theory, health care is often listed as one of the areas of "insurance or market failure" because competitive private markets have not been able to provide a sensible basis for comprehensive population coverage at an affordable level. Profits can usually only be made by restricting coverage to low-risk individuals, leaving those at higher risk uninsured or covered only by minimal public plans; or by limiting coverage to eligible services. Competitive insurance markets, like all markets, work to shift the risk, so that those most in need are more or less uninsurable. The whole idea of "pooling risk" through the community rating of a common public-payer structure is one key method to ensure that those most in need do get service. In this way, the burden of cost for those services is not borne by the poor and the unhealthy, but rather progressively distributed according to income.

SOCIALIZED MEDICINE OR POOLED RISK?

One occasionally hears that Canada has a "clumsy, state-run" system and that competitive insurance markets would make it more "efficient and modern," or that privately purchased health care would provide more choice for citizens and therefore we should allow it. As we stated in Chapter 2, in making this argument people fail to distinguish the three dimensions—financing, allocation, and delivery—of health care. When we separate out the dimensions, the fallacies of privatized health care become clear. First of all it's worth restating that almost all health care in Canada is already privately provided, although largely (but not exclusively) by not-for-profit providers. What we think of as public hospitals are in fact corporations, and the doctors, nurses, and other staff are not public servants, but employees whose conditions of employment are largely governed by the policies of those institutions and their independent boards. In most big cities, the large numbers of physicians and hospitals allow them to compete for patients. Canada already enjoys a very strong and unique partnership between the public and private sectors in the provision of its health services. A number of steps have been taken in many provinces to actually increase private managerial expertise by devolving the purchasing of health services to regional health authorities with professional management.

Canada's system is not state-run, but it is largely publicly financed. In Canada the state does not "run" our delivery system. It does not even have to run the payment function. This function could easily be performed by an independent and well-regulated agency. However, in order to pool risk in a progressive way, government revenues must be the major *source* of funds. The introduction of competitive private insurance markets for medically necessary health care would not fix our problems or relieve the burden on the publicly financed system. Instead, it would be tremendously divisive: the wealthy and the healthy would flock to private markets, leaving the sick and least able to pay in a second-rate public system. Competitive insurance markets would also introduce enormous overhead costs through higher administrative and advertising costs. As the world's outlier, only the U.S. persists in believing that competing markets in health insurance do anything other than add costs and reduce coverage.

WON'T MORE PRIVATE MONEY RELIEVE PRESSURE ON THE PUBLIC SYSTEM?

There is a common and intuitive notion that if people were allowed to purchase health care privately, it would free up resources in the public system and *strengthen* the public system by providing more public resources for those who cannot buy their services privately. On the face of it, this seems like a compelling story. However, appearances are misleading and the real-world effects of taking this approach have been quite different. Most studies have found a combination of higher costs and poorer access (longer waiting lists) whenever mixed-funding (public and private sources) models are introduced. How can this be true? It's counter-intuitive. It is true because, among other things, privately financed health services *require* as a market condition that the public system be inadequate or at least be perceived as inadequate, in order to make a private market compelling and viable. Otherwise why else would people choose to buy equivalent private services rather than get public services free.[4]

Rather than strengthening the public system, multi-tier models require a weak public system in order to make a tiered model supportable. In their recent report on private cataract surgery in Alberta, the Consumer Association of Canada concluded the following: contrary to commonly held beliefs and claims made by suppliers, the growth of private cataract surgery in Alberta has *increased* public waiting lists since the same physician works in both systems; *increased* the cost of services to the publicly financed plan, the direct costs to patients, and the cost of the health plan to the community at large; created a number of *conflicts of interest* jeopardizing taxpayers and patients; and *decreased* public accountability, scrutiny, and control of the Alberta provincial health insurance plan.[5] The consumers' report found that patients who paid privately were being charged up to $1,500 out-of-pocket. They were also being encouraged to purchase "better materials." Similar results have been found in Manitoba, Australia, and New Zealand.

It is important for private business to understand the costs associated with a private tier of health care since, as employers, they will likely be the ones who must pay for private insurance through employee benefits. As Bob Evans, one of Canada's distinguished health economists, reminds us, private business can be divided into two sets of interests with respect to health care: the vendors or sellers of health care whose product is and whose profits emanate from health care; and the business purchasers of health care, whose products range from cars to food to services, but who purchase health care on behalf of their employees through supplementary insurance benefit plans. Although *vendors* of health services sometimes present themselves as representing private business interests, it is the *purchasers* of health care services—most small, medium, and large companies—who bear the costs. This is why thoughtful Canadian corporate leaders like Red Wilson for Bell Canada Enterprises (BCE) recognize that lower health care costs in Canada represent a competitive advantage for Canadian business.[6]

The idea that competitive private insurers can somehow keep costs down flies in the face of what we know to be true in other areas: that a single payer/purchaser, a so-called monopsony purchaser, can drive much tougher bargains, and can insist that providers of care keep their costs down, since there is no one else for the providers to sell their services to: if insurers were competing for business they would have to offer higher prices to the same service providers or miss out. Anyone who is not sure of this should ask publishers if Chapters or Chapters/Indigo drive a hard bargain for bulk purchasing! Interestingly enough, American Health Management Organizations are learning this. As the larger HMOs buy up the smaller ones and become the only game in town, they are driving down their costs by negotiating tougher bargains with their medical employees and with pharmaceutical companies.

BUT DOCTORS IN CANADA ARE NOT ALLOWED TO OPT OUT OF THE PUBLIC SYSTEM, ARE THEY?

Critics have accused "the Canadian model" of being a health care system in which doctors are dependent employees who cannot practise outside of the public system.[7] They also assert that Canadians cannot buy health care privately. As we have already noted, hospital-based physicians and health care workers are *not* employees of the state, nor are doctors who practise in the community.

TABLE 3 – 1
Provincial Variations in Regulation of Privately-Financed Hospital and Physican Services

POLICY ISSUE	B.C.	ALTA.	SASK.	MAN.	ONT.	QUE.	N.B.	N.S.	P.E.I.	NFLD.
OPTING OUT OF PUBLIC INSURANCE PLAN										
Can physicians opt out of the public plan?	y (yes)	y	y	y	y	y	y	y	y	y
Can opted-in physicians bill patients directly?	n (no)[1]	y	y	n	n	n[1]	y	n	y	n
EXTRA-BILLING MEASURES										
Direct Prohibition: Is there an explicit ban on extra billing for opted-in physicians?	y[2]	y[2]	y	y	y	y	n[3]	y	n[3]	y[2]
Can opted-out physicians bill any amount?	y[2]	y[2]	y	n	n	y	y	n	y	y
Status Disincentive: Is public-sector coverage denied to patients receiving insured services from opted-out physicians?	y	y[2]	n[4]	n[4]	n[4]	y	y	n[4]	n	n[5]
PRIVATE INSURANCE FOR PUBLICLY-INSURED SERVICES										
Are contracts of private insurance for publicly insured services prohibited?	y	y	n	y	y	y	n	n	y	n
Can private insurance pay for all or part of an opted-out physician's fees?	n	n	y	n	n	n	y[6]	y[7]	n	y[5]

1 British Columbia and Quebec permit direct billing by opted-in physicians who make revocable election to do so; until they revoke the election they may not receive payment from the public plan.

2 Some exceptions allowed.

3 New Brunswick and Prince Edward Island have no specific ban on extrabilling, but rather rely on the elimination of public cross-subsidization of private service. In particular, they deny public coverage for patients receiving publicly insured services from physicians charging more than the fee set by the public plan.

4 Manitoba, Nova Scotia, and Ontario use neither status disincentive nor public subsidy elimination measures, relying solely on direct prohibition of extra-billing by opted-out physicians.

5 Newfoundland uses neither status nor price disincentives to deter extrabilling by opted-out physicians, and permits private insurance coverage for a top-up of public coverage for insured services rendered by them.

6 New Brunswick voids public coverage where any private insurance payment is received.

7 In Nova Scotia an opted-out physician can only charge privately up to the fee set in the public sector.

Is there something that bans doctors from selling private medical services? No is the short answer. Can doctors bill their patients directly? Can doctors charge more for services than the government will pay? The answer is, mostly, yes. It depends on which province you live in.

Table 3–1 highlights the variations in the kind of private charges that are allowed across the ten provinces in conformity with the CHA.

First, in order to understand this table, we need to define some terms: "Provincial Plan" refers to the health care plan run by the province that pays for health care. "Opted-in physicians" are doctors who have elected to practise within the provincial health care plan and be paid the fee agreed upon by the government and the medical association. "Opted-out physicians" are doctors who have elected to practise outside the provincial plan and bill patients directly for their services. As we can see from Table 3–1, physicians can practise outside the provincial plans, *in all provinces.* Canadians can buy services privately from these doctors if they wish. The fact that this does not happen often is a measure of how well the public system works.

Every province allows licensed doctors to choose whether they wish to practise within the provincial plan and be paid by the province, or outside the plan and be paid directly by their patients. If physicians decide they wish to opt out of the provincial plan, they give up their right to bill the plan directly for services they provide to their patients. The consequences of opting out differ from province to province.

Do doctors have to decide for all time whether they want to practise within the public plan or outside of it? That is, can they change their minds? The simple answer is yes, again. Doctors can and do change their minds. Licensed doctors who want to be paid from the provincial plan apply for a billing number. In exchange for the privilege of not worrying about collecting money from patients, they agree to the terms and conditions of the plan. If they decide they want to opt out, they surrender their billing number.

If doctors who decide to practise within the provincial plan are guaranteed payment for their services by the government, why would any doctor want to practise outside of the provincial plan? In all provinces except Manitoba, Nova Scotia, and Ontario, doctors who have opted out of the provincial plans can bill their patients whatever they want. When doctors charge a patient more than the fee that has been deemed appropriate for the service under the public plan, this is referred to as "extra-billing."

The Canada Health Act does not prohibit extra-billing by doctors who decide they want to be paid by the provincial plan, that is, doctors who have opted in. Rather it penalizes the provincial plan that allows such practices. If a province allows its opted-in doctors to bill more than the fee allowed by the provincial plan, then the federal government can deduct some of the money it transfers to the provinces for health care—one dollar for every dollar that the province allows a doctor to charge over the provincial plan. But, once again, how the provinces prohibit extra-billing differs from one province to another. In some provinces, extra-billing by opted-in doctors is out-and-out prohibited. In fact, all provinces except PEI and New Brunswick prohibit extra-billing by any physicians who also bill the provincial plan.

Yet even among those provinces that explicitly prohibit extra-billing, some (Alberta, British Columbia, and Newfoundland) allow exceptions. For example, an opted-in physician may charge extra for materials or equipment related to a publicly insured service if he or she can show that they were necessary in order to provide the service.

How does the provincial government enforce the provincial laws prohibiting opted-in doctors from charging above the amount stipulated in the plan? Opted-in physicians who do extra-bill are subject to a number of penalties, including fines, suspension from the provincial plan, and even disciplinary action by the professional regulatory body. For example, physicians in Alberta are fined $1,000 for the first offence and $2,000 for the second and subsequent offences.

What about New Brunswick and PEI? Do they allow doctors who have opted-in to the provincial plan to charge more than the plan? These provinces don't explicitly prohibit extra-billing. However, they will not pay these doctors the portion of the fee that the public plan funds. The patient, therefore, has to pay the *entire* fee, not only the extra amount, out of his or her own pocket. As a result, not many people would choose to go to a physician who charges more than the plan.

What about doctors who have opted out of the provincial plans entirely? Can they charge whatever they want? Yes and no, depending on the province they practise in. Manitoba, Nova Scotia, and Ontario prohibit opted-out physicians from charging more privately than the public plan would pay. In other words, if the public plan pays $100 for a medical checkup, the opted-out physician in these three provinces can charge no more than $100. Moreover, in Ontario, patients don't have to pay an opted-out physician for services they have received until they are reimbursed by the public plan.

In the other seven provinces, *opted-out physicians can charge whatever they wish.* Again there are a couple of exceptions. In Alberta, opted-out physicians cannot charge above the plan's fee schedule for services provided in an emergency. In British Columbia, opted-out doctors cannot extra-bill for services they provide in public hospitals or community care facilities.

If opted-out doctors in the other seven provinces can charge whatever they want, why don't more doctors in those provinces decide to opt-out of the public plan? In six of the seven provinces where opted-out doctors can extra-bill, the provinces discourage extra-billing through the elimination of public cross subsidization; opted-out physicians can charge any fee they want, but their patients will not be covered by the public plan for these services. In other words, if you, as a doctor, choose to opt out of the public plan and choose to bill more than the public plan allows, neither you nor your patient will be reimbursed for those services from the public plan.

Only Newfoundland will allow doctors to opt out, charge over the amount in the public plan and also pay the amount covered by the plan for that service. The patient is responsible for paying the extra amount.

If all provinces, except Newfoundland, refuse to pay anything to opted-out physicians who charge more than the public plan allows for insured medical services, why couldn't Canadians buy private insurance as they do in the U.S. and pay an opted-out doctor directly? Some provinces indeed specifically prohibit private insurance for services covered by the public plan. However, New Brunswick, Newfoundland, and Saskatchewan do not prohibit private insurance for all or part of the costs of opted-out physicians' services. As a result, in these three provinces, there may be opportunities for physicians to practise outside the plan, charge whatever they wish, and have their fees paid by private insurance. It is most likely, however, that provincial governments would move to prohibit private markets for medically necessary services.

If doctors can practise outside the health care system and, in some provinces, bill more than the fee the public plan pays, why don't more doctors do it? Part of the answer is simple economics. By deciding to practise within the public system, they have guaranteed payment for their services, without any of the private overhead required to recover on unpaid bills or the unproductive bureaucratic overhead of endless private insurance forms and prior approvals. No more bad cheques from patients. No more having to decide whether to deny care to someone who can't pay or to provide the service for free.

But that is not the only reason. Most doctors, as Canadians or residents of Canada, accept the fundamental system of values that has been part of the health care system from the beginning. They believe that everyone, regardless of their ability to pay, should get the same kind of health care—the best health care available. They believe that there should not be one kind of health care reserved for the rich (the best care) and one kind for the poor (whatever is left). They believe that you should not be able to buy your way to the front of the line for care, that care should be given first to those who are the sickest and need it most. Indeed, despite pressures from a minority of physicians to recommend the introduction of private financing into our system, the Canadian Medical Association has consistently supported a publicly financed single-payer system.

Isn't there a problem of sustainability of our public system?

We hear talk of "sustainability" and, given the tremendous pressures experienced in the health care sector in the last decade from the fiscal squeeze of the mid-nineties, the worry seems a valid one. There is concern about the capacity of the public treasury to "sustain" our system. But we noted earlier, Canada actually reduced spending on health care in the mid-nineties; growth in the late

1990s began to pick up again as the economy became more robust. So it is a bit of a leap to say that public spending is not sustainable when we have just displayed a remarkable feat of cost control. Health spending in Canada is currently well within the line of spending as in other, comparable industrialized countries.

In fact, based on work by the Conference Board of Canada using national expenditure information, average annual real per capita growth in health expenditures (adjusted for inflation and population growth) throughout the 1990s was there, but quite modest, reflecting decisions by governments to reign in public spending. Real growth in total expenditure was a modest 1.6 percent, public expenditure was 1.2 percent, and private expenditure was 2.5 percent.

Figure 3–1 illustrates this real growth in total per capita health spending in Canada in 5-year intervals over the last two decades. It shows the actual reduction in public spending in the 1990-1995 period when governments were reigning in spending to control debt and the rebound growth in the 1995-2000 period. Overall spending

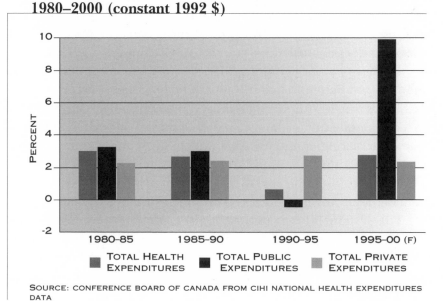

FIGURE 3-1

Real Per Capita Total, Public and Private Health Expenditures 5-Year Annual Growth Rates, Canada, 1980–2000 (constant 1992 $)

TOTAL HEALTH EXPENDITURES

TOTAL PUBLIC EXPENDITURES

TOTAL PRIVATE EXPENDITURES

SOURCE: CONFERENCE BOARD OF CANADA FROM CIHI NATIONAL HEALTH EXPENDITURES DATA

in the last decade and the last five years has remained at levels consistent with growth in the last two decades. Far from spending being "out of control," overall spending has remained relatively constant over the last two decades, and the most effective spending control was managed by governments under intense fiscal pressure.

The limitations on sustainability for a high-quality health care system, we would argue, are more political than fiscal. Our economy is reasonably solid and governments, having largely balanced their operating budgets, are beginning to retire debt. There is room for modest growth in the health care sector in both the public and private sides of health care in Canada, and polls indicate that Canadians show a greater willingness to invest public money in health care than in any other public service.

You may argue that this approach is fine for now, but what about the future? There is concern that the aging of the population will send health care costs through the roof, and that these costs will be felt most directly when the baby boomers enter the final years of their lives. On the contrary, although the elderly are likely to place greater demands on health care resources, much of the careful analysis suggests that health service use by the elderly adjusts with the available public resources.[8] There is some reason to be encouraged that health service use in the older population is a reflection of the "compression of morbidity"—the fact that the elderly are actually healthier than they used to be.[9] A simple forward linear projection on age-related spending does not take these realities into account.

The costs of an aging population are likely to be less critical than the absolute number and mix of health care workers and professionals, the way they are organized into care teams, and the way we compensate them—how we pay doctors, and at what level. These questions are generating considerable interest and attention across Canada, and a number of pilot programs have been set up to test ideas for reform in the area of financing of primary-care services for general family practice doctors and some nurse-practitioners.

The sustainability argument is also raised because health care spending is growing and as a proportion of provincial spending, it may soon account for 50 percent of provincial spending in some provinces. *Hello!* For forty years health spending has been growing as a proportion of provincial resources. While it may well be worth asking whether health care spending always yields the best return on health improvements in the population, there is nothing intrinsically alarming about the share of provincial spending on health care. Indeed, health care and education have become the biggest-ticket items for provincial governments in Canada, and they will continue to be. It is certainly true that as health care consumes a greater portion of provincial spending, it will become increasingly politicized since it will become more and more what government is about.

The sustainability argument is often raised when the political agenda of tax reductions collides with prudent public funding on health care. However, those are separate issues: it is one thing to push an agenda of tax reduction and another to argue that public spending is unsustainable, especially when we have actually done a very good job of controlling costs. This specious "sustainability" argument is sometimes a rhetorical way of advancing another agenda—an argument in favour of more "private" money, based on the question of sustainability, is one way to alter who pays and who benefits, in favour of those with greater means.

Enlarging the share of private payment might well have the effect of reducing public spending levels, but it would not help to control overall costs. Moreover, it would be a departure and, in our view, a step backward from notions of solidarity and risk pooling.

The fact is that privately financed services are usually more expensive. When a patient visits a privately paid physiotherapist in Ontario, he or she (or the private insurance carrier) usually pays two to three times what a provincial health insurance plan pays that physiotherapist for identical treatment. When cancer patients from Ontario travel to the U.S. for radiation treatment, as they have done recently, the costs in the U.S. are as much as six times as high as they would be in Canada. Would someone please explain how it can be cheaper to introduce privately insured services into Canada if services are to be two to six times the cost?

The only honest conclusion to this question is that competitive private health insurance can be made cheaper *only if fewer and less sick people get insured*, fewer services are covered, or limitations are placed on the amount of service. This option is acceptable only if we abandon the risk pooling and progressive tax elements of Canada's system. This is precisely what is going on in the U.S. at this moment. The numbers of the uninsured and underinsured are large, eligibility criteria for coverage are stricter, fewer services are covered, and caps on services have been introduced. And the U.S. system is still the most expensive and inefficient in the world.

To allow a mixed funding system and still ensure comprehensive coverage for everyone *will* cost Canadian society more than it currently does. As Professor Raisa B. Deber notes, "If we as a society cannot afford care within the publicly funded sector, we certainly cannot afford it privately."[10] Or perhaps more to the point, the sick will not be able to afford it. A mixed financing system will only work if we are prepared to deny care to those who cannot afford to pay for it privately.

WOULDN'T USER FEES DISCOURAGE ABUSE?

A common "zombie idea" (or meme that refuses to die despite evidence to its worthlessness) in health care is that a small charge would deter unnecessary use and add more money to the system.[11] Once again, at first glance, this makes a lot of sense. Considerable research has shown, however, that the desired result is not exactly what occurs. The underlying assumption in the argument is that people are frivolous and seek treatment when it is not needed. While this may have some truth to it, user fees have a perverse, unintended effect. They do reduce utilization under some circumstances, but the research demonstrates that they reduce both unnecessary *and* necessary visits, indiscriminately. And even low charges are much better at deterring visits from the poor (who usually have poorer health) than visits from the wealthy.

A number of jurisdictions have user fees. Mr. Chrétien recently remarked on this in regard to Sweden. We would note that in most European jurisdictions, user fees are a tiny portion of health care insurance that is often more comprehensive than Canada's. Indeed, in most jurisdictions in Europe that have user fees, the fees exist within a much broader social insurance context than that in Canada.

As we noted previously in our hamburger examples, the amount of actual demand in the health care system is the subject of much dispute. At a minimum we can say that most health expenditures can be identified as physician-initiated events. Individuals may make the first decision to see a doctor, but subsequent visits are largely scheduled and set up by the doctor or at his or her suggestion. All of the most costly decisions require a doctor's interventions: admission to hospital, drug prescriptions, surgery, radiotherapy, and more intrusive events. To be effective, user fees would have to deter the patients from going to the doctor in the first place.

The deterring of unnecessary visits as well as necessary ones usually results in more expensive care when the patient deteriorates. Careful analysis also suggests that avoidable complications from related conditions such as diabetes, hypertension, and so on also increase when care is deterred. In the U.S. many of the poorest members of the population only find they are victims of disease late in their diseased state, at which time they face expensive hospitalization that may have been prevented by earlier treatment. In Quebec, user fees for prescription drugs in the elderly resulted in increased hospital admissions and complications from untreated disease.[12]

As health policy analysts have known for some time, the easiest way to contain costs is to shift them to somebody else. User fees shift costs away from governments to the patient, but they end up increasing the overall cost to society. To contain their own costs, governments have an incentive to shift them outside the publicly paid system; this results in what has been called "passive privatization." This shifting is being documented in the areas of home care and in pharmaceuticals and is beginning to occur in the rehabilitation area as well. What we must remember is that whether care is paid for publicly or privately individual Canadians foot the bill. The difference is that in a publicly financed health care system, care is provided on the basis of need rather than on the ability to pay and costs are distributed according to the ability to pay.

In case we have not said it enough, the key challenges in Canada are not with the financing mechanism; they are with the allocation or purchasing mechanism, the delivery and management of services, and in updating the range of services we publicly cover. Canadian health care financing is one thing Canada has done right. We have to find new ways of making better use of our relatively effective payment mechanism, revitalize our management and delivery systems and allow the extension of public coverage to areas not currently provided for through the Canada Health Act.

Canaries in the Mine: Waiting for Care

Canadians want their health care system to respond to them accord-ing to their needs.[1] This means that equal needs will be treated equally and unequal needs will be treated differentially. Those most in need, as in an emergency situation, ought to be moved to the front of the line. A system that fails to ensure that people get care in the order of relative need or urgency would be viewed by many Canadians as inherently unfair and cause for concern. As eminent Canadian health researchers have stated, "In a publicly financed health system, waiting is among other things a measure of distribu-tive justice."[2]

Waiting for specialist and hospital services has become a major flashpoint of public concern about our health care system across the country. Scenes of hundreds of cancer patients being bussed to bor-der cities for radiation therapy and patients being turned away from emergency rooms have properly captured the public interest in Canada and require better responses than we have had to date. There is an outcry and calls for increased funding to deal with the situation.[3] Waiting lists and waiting times have also become key points of argument for those who would like to introduce private competitive insurance reform.

Are waiting lists like canaries in a mine? As canaries warn (by their death) that there is no oxygen in the mine, are waiting lists an indication of a system coming apart at the seams? Are they akin to the canary in the mine? Is waiting always worse than not waiting? The short answer is not always. We need to understand the nature and causes of waiting lists and do a better job at managing them. However, part of the difficulty in answering these questions and understanding the problem is the lack of standardized definitions and measurements of waiting. A large research team commissioned by Health Canada a few years ago to study the issue of waiting times concluded that "with rare exceptions waiting lists in Canada, as in most countries, are non-standardized, capriciously organized, poorly monitored and (according to most informed observers) are in grave need of retooling."[4] As such, most of the lists currently being publicized are at best misleading sources of data on access to care and at worst mischievous misinformation propaganda.

To come up with meaningful solutions to wait times, we need to speak the same language and measure the same thing. To restore confidence in Canadian health care the public needs to understand this issue. More important, it is necessary for Canadians to understand that to attempt to ease waiting lists by allowing people to purchase care privately is misguided. It is a false promise. It will not work.

WHAT IS A WAITING LIST AND HOW IS IT MEASURED?

We need to begin the discussion with some definitions before we can understand the nature of the problem. A *waiting list*, or *wait list*, for health care is a list of patients awaiting a surgical, medical, or diagnostic procedure or an appointment with a professional, such as a specialty care physician. A *waiting time* or *wait time*, is the amount of time a patient is on a waiting list before receiving a medical, surgical, or diagnostic procedure.

Most waiting lists are kept by individual physicians. With the exception of some cancer registries and cardiac care networks, there is no overarching manager of these diverse lists, and astonishingly little coordination of waiting list information across sites and across specialty care areas among physicians. Whether it is appropriate for a patient to be on a list is largely the decision of an individual physician. There are *few* agreed-upon rules for when a patient should be placed on a list. As a result, physicians differ in their decisions as to who to place on a list, and when. Sometimes wait lists may be inflated by an individual physician because longer lists indicate that he or she is in greater demand and, therefore, must be good. As a result, waiting lists, rather than measuring unmet need, may more accurately reflect unmet demand by providers. This is less surprising than you might think, given that physicians are paid to look after individual patients, not populations of patients.

The accuracy of waiting lists is affected by a number of factors. Lists are not usually audited to see if patients' needs or wishes have changed. Some patients are placed on a list inappropriately, some are on more than one list for the same procedure, some have already received the procedure, some don't even know they are on a list and, rarely, some have died before receiving a procedure. As a result, the number of people on a list is not meaningful without information on how long they have been on the list, the urgency of their condition relative to other patients on the list, whether they are on the list appropriately, and what the usual/recommended wait is.

To demonstrate the importance of understanding how data are collected and their validity, let's look at two sets of results: one from the Fraser Institute and one from the Manitoba Centre for Health Policy and Evaluation at the University of Manitoba. The Fraser Institute, using surveys of physicians' opinions, publishes an annual report on how long a patient may expect to wait for a procedure. In 1999 the Fraser Institute reported that Canadians waited about 8.4 weeks between a specialist visit and a medical procedure, arguing a 15 percent increase from their 1998 survey.[5] The Fraser Institute also reported a 1999 waiting time of 7.2 weeks in Manitoba. Meanwhile, using actual medical and hospital encounter data, researchers at the Manitoba Centre found the real average wait time to be thirty days and bypass surgery waits to be shorter than the previous year![6] Two very different sets of results, which would lead to different conclusions and sets of solutions. Having well-managed information systems is a first step not only to managing access to care, but also to evaluating the performance of the delivery system.

As mentioned, wait time is the amount of time a patient is on a wait list before receiving the service. However, this can be calculated in different ways: retrospectively, cross-sectionally, or by prospective measurement. Without going into the differences between these measurements, suffice it to say that each method is employed to calculate different things and therefore gives different measures of waiting times. Moreover, none of these methods will necessarily answer the question most patients ask, "How long will I have to wait?"

Does a wait time start from the first onset of a patient's symptoms, the first appointment with the GP, the appointment with the specialty care practitioner, the first diagnostic test once a specialist has identified the patient as in need of a procedure, or from the time the procedure is booked? As is clear, depending on which starting point you use, the waiting time can vary in length. So when you hear or read that waiting times for breast cancer radiation is sixty days, you need more information before you get alarmed.

ARE WAITING LISTS AND WAITING TIMES TOO LONG IN CANADA?

The news that 5,000 people might be on a wait list would make for great newspaper headlines. However, if we learned that these people were on a wait list for a condition that is not life-threatening, and that the usual waiting time is about ten weeks, the news seems less disturbing. By contrast, breast or neck cancer patients who have been waiting too long and must be sent to the U.S. for quick treatments create real and justifiable concern. Likewise, although less dramatic, patients who have to wait for extended periods of time for cataract surgery—a simple procedure that creates an enormous improvement in the quality of life—also raise the spectre of the dying canary in the mine.

Before we can answer the question above, we need to be able to define what "too long" means. We need guidelines and protocols to reassure us about appropriate treatment times. We need to determine whether the problem is acute, short-lived or a chronic condition that has already existed for a long time. We need to develop consistent methods for deciding when patients should be put on lists and how to rank them in order of relative urgency. Their condition should be re-evaluated at standardized points; there should be guidelines for moving them from low to high priority as their condition changes and for removing them from the process entirely if their condition improves or they decide not to have the procedure. When we have standardized definitions and measurements we can begin to understand the underlying causes of waiting lists and times. Only with this understanding can we appropriately target solutions.

ADVERSE EFFECTS OF WAITING ON PATIENTS, PROVIDERS, AND THE HEALTH CARE SYSTEM

The fact is that lengthy wait times for medical services can have adverse effects on the quality of life for patients. This has been shown in studies of hip and knee replacements in Canada,[7] in other orthopedic procedures in the U.K.,[8] and also in prostate treatments[9] and cardiac bypass procedures.[10] In addition to quality-of-life issues, disease morbidity and the progression of the disease may worsen while the patient is waiting—although here the evidence is somewhat equivocal. For example, an audit of a British wait list discovered that 10 percent of the people waiting for cataract surgery had the potential for irreversible loss of vision.[11] In contrast, for others in the U.K., there were no demonstrable adverse consequences for delays in tonsil surgery[12] or urological surgery.[13]

With regard to the increased risks of death, a large Manitoba study concluded that urgent cardiovascular cases did receive relatively rapid surgery, and the non-urgent patients who had to wait showed no increased risk of death.[14] A similar conclusion was reached in Manitoba regarding cardiac catheterization.[15] In Ontario, in a review of the provincial patient registry for coronary bypass patients in 1991, less than 0.5 percent died while waiting and 3 people had surgery deferred after a non-fatal heart attack.[16] A comparable Halifax study of patients referred for bypass showed a very small (1.2 percent) mortality rate across four categories of urgency.[17] In those waiting for open heart surgery in Montreal, no effect on mortality was observed,[18] and these cardiovascular results are very similar to those reported elsewhere.[19,20,21] One must remember that inevitably some patients die even if they have received a procedure in a timely manner. So even in those few who died while waiting, death cannot be definitely attributed to the delay.

It appears then that waiting time for cardiac surgery, one of the most dangerous of medical waits, may not significantly alter mortality risk. This almost certainly reflects the increasing capacity of hospital admissions staff to triage intelligently and manage wait lists by level of urgency in order to avoid fatal outcomes. One would expect that lengthy waiting times for potentially curable malignancies would show a strong link with premature death, but though Canadian waiting times for radiation treatment are clearly high by international standards (which, incidentally, are only partially based on hard evidence), the precise impact on clinical outcomes of waiting for radiation remains unclear. A number of studies on cancer waiting times will shortly be published and will shed light on these important and sensitive waiting time and mortality relationships. However, whether waiting for radiation treatment causes premature mortality or not, it certainly adversely affects quality of life and confidence in our system, and we must do something to improve the situation.

Waiting is not uniformly bad. At times it is the patient's own choice. Sometimes a patient's condition spontaneously improves, and performing a procedure right away turns out to have been unnecessary; perhaps there's a painful operation, requiring recovery time, and costs to the health care system may be avoided. Sometimes patients appear to be waiting a long time, but that is only because their physicians put them on the list in anticipation that they might require a procedure, which in the end may or may not be necessary. Some people also appear to be waiting longer than others because they have already refused the procedure at an earlier opportunity for reasons arising out of their personal circumstances. Some patients also choose to wait so that they can seek other opinions or organize their lives.

Health care providers are also affected when their patients get on to lists and have to wait for periods of time. As keepers of lists, physicians often feel uncomfortable about making what are essentially economic decisions, rationing treatment while remaining responsible for the well-being of their patients. They are also frustrated by their inability to deliver what they perceive as optimal care, and worry about legal liabilities if waiting leads to complications.

Finally, long waiting lists, whether appropriate or not, have an impact on the well-being of the health care system. The strength of a publicly funded health care system is dependent on the confidence and willingness of the public to support it. Waiting, as we have stated, does not always pose significant risks to patients. However, the perception by the public that waiting lists are a problem is a *major* risk factor for our health care system. Waiting erodes the public's confidence that the Canadian health care system can still deliver the goods.

WHY ARE WAIT LISTS LONGER IN CANADA THAN IN THE U.S?

Wait lists are part of managing a publicly funded health care system. Systems of privately financed care require excess capacity to provide services in order to be competitive. Their ability to attract patients is based on the ready availability of technology and providers—so that they can boast of shorter or no waiting lines. However, systems with excess capacity are wasteful, inefficient, and more costly. There are long periods during which equipment, and personnel who must still be paid are idle. Publicly financed systems, however, typically do not carry excess capacity in either equipment or personnel. In order to keep costs down and make proper use of public funds, they try to ensure that supply matches demand so that equipment and personnel are both in constant use. As a result, care must be triaged on the basis of need: without excess capacity not everyone can be treated immediately. In this fashion our system tries to balance equity (access based on need, regardless of income) with efficiency (no waste) and accountability (appropriate use of public funds) among competing priorities.

Because the health care system is largely private and competitive in the United States, decisions about investment and training capacity are not coordinated or shared. Health organizations there have also built for peak load periods. As two Canadian health analysts put it, "The United States could be described as suffering from the side-effects of a medical equipment arms race."[22] Aside from opportunity costs of investing in technology that lies idle, there is now very good evidence, as we stated in Chapter 1, that many Americans receive inappropriate and unnecessary care, with adverse effects.[23]

The real scandal in the United States is that with surplus capacity and idle equipment, millions of Americans wait forever. Those who cannot afford to buy adequate insurance, or any insurance at all, do not receive adequate care. For these people, being on a waiting list in Canada could be considered a privilege.

It is worth noting (as we also did in Chapter 1) that crowding and diversion in emergency rooms are not problems limited to Canada; in fact, they are sometimes described as a nation-wide problem in the U.S.[24]

POTENTIAL CAUSES AND APPROPRIATE SOLUTIONS TO WAITING

There can be a number of different causes of long waiting lists and, therefore, different solutions to the problem. Is the underlying cause a human resource problem, poor working conditions and salaries, an overall shortage of personnel, geographic remoteness, quality-of-life issues, insufficiently trained personnel, inappropriate use of resources, or poor planning? Each cause leads to a different solution.

In some rural and remote areas, there may be shortages of particular types of professional providers, which produce long waits. Often governments will give financial incentives to providers to locate in these areas. But money is often not the problem. It may be that there are no appropriate jobs for the spouse or schools for their children. Sometimes on a fee-for-service payment schedule, physicians cannot make a decent income in some areas. In the latter instance, a different way of reimbursing physicians, such as some form of blended payment of fee-for-service and salary, might be helpful.

In some specialty care areas, like cancer care where the incidence of cancer is growing by 3 percent a year, the problem may be that there are not enough diagnostic or other machines or that personnel such as medical oncologists, physicists, and radiation therapy technicians are hard to find. The answer may be to train and recruit more professionals. However, if there is a shortage of machines, it is difficult to provide the clinical training for these students. Some provinces have resorted to recruiting from overseas. But in some of these disciplines there is a worldwide shortage of personnel. Overseas recruitment drives result in richer countries enticing workers from poorer countries—a brain drain that we ourselves have experienced with the U.S.

In determining solutions to wait lists, we need to know whether the problem is an acute problem or a chronic one. If we know, for example, that the problem in cancer radiation therapy is a shortage of providers, and we have addressed the issue through increased enrolment in training programs or aggressive recruitment, we can be confident that in a few years there will be sufficient numbers to provide the needed care. In such a situation, busing patients now to the U.S. might make good sense. With a little more investment, effective prevention, and screening programs, these supply problems in the field of cancer care will be historical events.

As we noted in Chapter 1, problems such as overcrowding in emergency rooms in many parts of North America over the last few winters and the rerouting of ambulances may have had more to do with the annual flu outbreak and physician practice patterns than any serious structural problems. The answer to date has been to provide more funding to hospitals so that they can hire more staff. There are two problems with this answer. As we know, there are problems with after-hours coverage for physicians' services as well as shortages of providers in some specialty areas and in some jurisdictions. Secondly, staffing hospitals for peak periods is wasteful. There are better solutions. Some jurisdictions—like Saskatchewan, Alberta, and, more recently, Ontario—have taken preventive measures, such as publicly providing flu vaccines for their populations. With good influenza inoculation programs, Sakatchewan and Alberta did not have the same emergency room crisis.[25] Alberta and Sakatchewan also have regional authorities that compel integration of emergency room services, whereas Ontario has struggled continuously to encourage co-operation between free-standing hospitals.

Money isn't always the answer

Attempts to reduce waiting lists by simply pouring money into the system do not appear to have worked very well.[26] Sometimes adding extra resources is counterproductive (this recently happened in the U.K.) because it produces what is known as a "feedback effect." When extra resources have been added to an area with long waiting lists, physicians increase their rate of referrals for that procedure, thereby offsetting any gains.[27]

About ten years ago Ontario successfully reduced coronary-artery bypass queues with the infusion of some new money and increased surgical volumes. However, the money and increased surgeries would not have been enough. Ontario also created a coordinated cardiac network, supported by an information system that allowed for auditing, monitoring, re-prioritizing of patients and co-ordination of access across all centres.

As stated earlier, the cause of the waiting must be examined to determine the appropriate solution. Simply adding money may not solve the problem. Worse still, those funds might have been used more appropriately elsewhere in the health care system, or in other areas such as additional supportive housing, reduced class sizes, and so on. We need good information on which to base such decisions, and we have to make careful choices amongst competing priorities.

WILL ALLOWING PATIENTS TO PURCHASE HOSPITAL OR MEDICAL SERVICES PRIVATELY HELP REDUCE WAITING LISTS AND TIMES?

The answer, according to evidence from natural international experiments, is apparently no. In the U.K. about 20 percent of all non-urgent heart surgery is done privately; the figure is comparable in New Zealand. The bulk of private surgical work focuses on hips, hernias, hemorrhoids, cataracts and gynecological procedures. Despite the opportunity to purchase these services privately, these are all conditions with some of the longest waiting times in the *public sector* in those jurisdictions. You might say that the waiting times in the public sector would be even longer without the option of private purchase. But, let's consider the international experience. In New Zealand, 37 percent of the population had supplementary private hospital insurance. In 1998, 21 percent of New Zealanders waited more than four months for elective surgery in the public system. In Australia the figures are 31.2 percent with supplementary insurance and 13 percent waiting longer than four months. In England the figures are 11.5 percent with supplementary private hospital insurance and 29 percent waiting longer than four months for elective procedures. In Canada, which effectively eliminates private medical or hospital insurance (supplementary private hospital insurance is limited to hotel services), less than 1.0 percent of Canadians were on wait lists, and fewer than 10 percent of those on wait lists waited longer than four months in 1998.[28] An apparent conclusion to these natural experiments in other jurisdictions is that the availability of private insurance is generally associated with *longer* wait times for patients in the public system. Allowing people to buy medical and hospital care privately does not reduce waiting time in the public system.

Let's explore this further with a Canadian example. Keep in mind that the presence of the more expensive private option is only viable when the public option is inadequate. Otherwise, why would patients choose to pay for services from their own pockets if the public system can provide them with timely, high quality care? When providers are allowed to work in both the public and private systems simultaneously, they often inform their patients that if they see them in their private clinic they can perform the procedure more quickly than in the public clinic. From the physician's perspective, this makes good economic sense, since in many countries a physician gets more for services in the private clinic. Although, in three provinces in Canada, physicians may only be entitled to the same fee in the private facility as they would receive in the public one, they are able to increase their incomes by persuading patients to purchase extra private services, "better" quality materials, and so on.

FIGURE 4 - 1

Median Waiting Time for Cataract Surgery in Manitoba 1998/1999

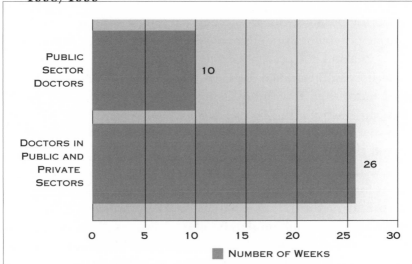

SOURCE: MANITOBA CENTRE FOR HEALTH POLICY AND EVALUATION

We noted in Chapter 3 that, according to the Consumer Association of Alberta, the growth of private cataract surgery has increased public waiting lists. Similar results occurred in Manitoba, where until 1999 ophthalmologists could operate in either the public system alone or in both the public and the private systems. Work by the Manitoba Centre for Health Policy and Evaluation in 1998 and 1999 showed an unusual and perhaps not surprising trend. The average wait time for cataract surgery for physicians who operate only in the public sector was ten weeks. For physicians operating in both the private and public systems the average waiting time on their *public* list was twenty-six weeks! Apparently long wait lists in the public system increase demand for speciality services in the more lucrative private system. The success of a private payment option is thus dependent on the market requirement that the public tier perform poorly! This suggests that a parallel private tier does what it is supposed to do: provide faster access for those with deeper pockets, a development that sometimes does compromise access for those waiting in the public system.[29]

This experience of high public waits in Canada in areas with high levels of private insurance has also been documented in Britain.[30]

WAITING AND DISTRIBUTIVE JUSTICE

As we explained earlier, wait lists are one way of managing resources effectively and efficiently in publicly financed systems or systems with finite resources. The question is: how do we manage wait lists to ensure fairness in accessing services? As Lewis and Sanmartin[31] outline, fairness can be achieved in one of four ways: randomness (patients are chosen to receive services by chance or lottery); desert or merit (patients are chosen on the basis of some individual characteristic unrelated to their health status, such as income or education); order of presentation (first come, first served); or condition (patients are chosen on the basis of their relative medical need or prospect to benefit). All four methods are "fair," in that they either exhibit no bias or the rules for ordering are transparent and agreed upon; however, all but the last one separate access from need. One of the reasons Canadians came up with a universal, publicly funded health system in the first place is that we believe the distribution of health services should be based on need, and not on chance, being the early bird, being richer, or some other characteristic unrelated to health.

As we demonstrated earlier, being allowed to purchase care privately is apparently *not* only about patient choice or reducing costs. It is about distributing health resources according to something other than health need or the ability to benefit. It is about allocating resources based on criteria inversely related to health needs, i.e., wealth.

However, decisions about allocating finite resources, either to individuals according to need or across different program areas, require transparent information and management tools. A number of projects within Canada have been experimenting with wait-list management tools.

CURRENT INITIATIVES IN CANADA

In the field of cancer, Cancer Care Ontario has taken a number of steps to reduce waiting lists and times. It has launched a major effort that has eliminated referrals to the U.S. by launching a large after-hours clinic to increase services (www.cancercare.on.ca/news/12jan2001.html) and by recruiting close to ninety new radiation therapists in the last year to increase the volume of patients who can get radiation treatment. This initiative has drawn fire from critics because a private, for-profit clinic has been running the after-hours service. Even with the additional charges of the private clinic, the public is absorbing the charges without fees for individual patients.

While this may deal with backlogs, efforts must also be made to co-ordinate and manage lists better. Where waiting-list data are carefully and accurately compiled, routinely monitored, and used to co-ordinate timely access, the public clearly benefits.

The Cardiac Care Network of Ontario, which is funded by the provincial government, ensures timely access to cardiac surgery and some ambulatory procedures through a set of consensus guidelines for allocating services to patients on the basis of clinical priority. It is widely viewed as a model approach to the coordination of access to cardiac care among specialists and across the province. In March

2000, Ontario also announced a joint-replacement wait-list coordination initiative modelled on the Cardiac Care Network. The other major initiative is the Western Canada Wait List (WCWL) Project (www.wcwl.org), funded by the federal government's Health Transition Fund. Nineteen partners in the four western provinces, including regional health authorities, medical associations, provincial ministries of health and health research centres are testing a priority ranking system, based on urgency, across five clinical areas, including MRI scanning, cataract surgery, orthopedic procedures, pediatric mental health services, and general surgery. Point-counting tools, scored by physicians, for assigning priority to patients on waiting lists, were developed through extensive clinical input from multidisciplinary clinical panels. These tools have been implemented, evaluated, and modified accordingly. The WCWL Project has just issued its final report. Overall, the researchers found that the priority-setting tools were useful and valid and had won support from providers, regional health authorities, and the public. This initiative provides us with accurate information and fair, agreed-upon criteria for determining who gets care, and when, in the five clinical areas. These tools will not only improve the fairness and effectiveness of the care provided, they also allow us to monitor the effectiveness of services within a clinical area and, ultimately, to compare the effectiveness of care across clinical areas. However, the WCWL project is just a beginning; it needs to be extended across the country and across clinical areas.

CONCLUSION

The first requirement for dealing with waiting lists is to develop better information systems based on standardized definitions and measurements that provide real-time, useful information for health decision makers and for patients. The development of priority-setting tools for the monitoring and evaluation of people on waiting lists is essential to improve fairness, effectiveness and efficiency of services. However, waiting-list management for specific procedures or conditions may affect access to services and resource allocation in other areas and, therefore, is just the beginning. We need to be able to prioritize across different clinical procedures and across the health system in its entirety in order to allocate resources to those service areas that will produce the best health outcomes for the population. Without such a common framework, inequities are likely to develop over time. As Lewis and Sanmartin[32] indicate, we already cross-prioritize, but the rules are implicit, unarticulated, and lacking in transparency. Explicit cross-prioritization requires commonly accepted and valid indicators of need and prospects for benefit from care. That this will be difficult goes without saying. But, as stated above, the status quo is neither efficient nor effective, and it must be reformed.

Waiting lists and waiting times are areas in which public concern about the system is extremely high. The restoration of public confidence requires immediate action. Over the next few years we must attack the problem of waiting lists vigorously and intelligently. This will require accurate assessment of the evidence and the careful engagement of motivated health care leaders, and professionals, managers and funders (government), to accelerate the management of our waiting lists.

Closer to Home and Out of Pocket: Shifting Sites of Care

With hospital restructurings and closures in the last decade, medical and technical advancements, and the public preference for remaining in their own homes, health care has been moving out of institutions and into the community.[1] The home and home care are becoming the new frontiers for health care

This shift in the site of care has also been fuelled by governments' concern about the increasing demand and need for health care as the population ages. Higher life expectancies have made the elderly a growing population. In 1995, there were an estimated 3.6 million seniors in Canada, representing 12 percent of the total population, up from 10 percent in 1981. In 1998, 12.3 percent of the Canadian population was 65 and over.[2, 3] Compared to European countries Canada still has a relatively young population, but Statistics Canada projections to the year 2026 show that while the Canadian population will grow at an average rate of 0.6 percent each year over the next twenty-six years, the population over the age of 65 will increase at an average rate of 2.7 percent per year. This suggests that, by the year 2016, 21.5 percent of Canadians will be older than 65 and more than 5 percent will be over 80. This increase in the elderly will have implications for home care costs and for the total amount of money Canadians will pay for health care, including the amount they will pay directly out of their own pockets.

WHAT IS HOME CARE?

Some provinces refer to the service as "long-term care," others "continuing care," and yet others "home care." In some provinces long-term care (LTC) services refer to residential care (nursing homes) for the elderly or people with chronic disabilities, and home care refers to health and social services provided in the home and community. In other provinces (Ontario for example) LTC services refer both to care provided in the community or home and to residential care.

Home care encompasses an array of services that enable clients who are incapacitated in whole or in part to live at home, often with the effect of preventing, delaying, or substituting residential or acute care alternatives.[4] Home care can sometimes also refer to social services based in the community, but coordinated through home care programs. Home care can be required for a long term, but it can also be necessary for a short period of time.

Home care services are typically those provided in people's homes. They include professional care (for example, nursing, physiotherapy, occupational therapy, speech therapy), personal supports (for example, bathing and toileting), and homemaking (cleaning, laundry, meal preparation); they may include respite services, medical supplies, equipment programs, and palliative care. Community support services include meals-on-wheels, transportation, security checks, friendly visiting and adult day programs. There are also Alzheimer's community programs and supportive living programs.

Originally, home care was thought of as a bundle of services required by the elderly or by adults and children with chronic disabilities in order to allow them to live in the home for as long as possible. However, the home care population has always included some acute-care patients released from hospitals who still require after care (such as changing of bandages). This group of "step-down" clients has been increasing in the last decade as more acute care can be provided outside of hospitals and patients are released earlier and sicker from hospitals. As a result, home care programs are now treating more clients with significantly higher levels of acute illness than in the past.

Improved technologies are also changing the scope and delivery of home care in Canada. Although it was unheard-of twenty years ago, it is now not unusual for clients to receive intravenous therapy, nutrition therapy, hydration, antibiotics, chemotherapy, or pain control in their homes. Other technology-intensive therapies include renal and peritoneal dialysis. There is more complex ventilator care, especially for children, more central-line infusion treatment, more patient-controlled analgesia pumps, and different types of post-surgical care (especially with more same-day surgery in hospitals, including back surgeries, mastectomies, replacement of arthritic joints, and so on). Other advances have been made with drug therapy over the last five years, including dramatic advances in thrombolytic treatment.

Because of these different populations, home care can be thought of as having three functions: maintenance (allowing clients to stay independent in their current living environment instead of having to move to a more expensive situation), prevention (services and monitoring, which over time lead to overall lower costs of care and an improved quality of life for clients), and substitution (services that are provided in hospitals and long term care facilities, but can also be provided in the home).

Home care is both publicly and privately funded. Professional services such as nursing, rehabilitation therapy, and nutritional services are usually funded by government. In addition, governments often pay in full or in part for homemaking services if they are required in order for the client to remain in the home. Other services such as respite services, meals programs, transportation, medical equipment and supplies involve user fees tied to income. Which services are subject to user fees and how much and how they are determined varies across the country. The way in which these services are delivered also varies across the country.

Services are provided by public, not-for-profit, for-profit, and volunteer agencies. In Saskatchewan, Quebec, PEI, Yukon, Northwest Territories, and Nunavut, professional and home support services are delivered mainly by employees of publicly funded agencies. In New Brunswick, Newfoundland, British Columbia and Alberta all professional services are delivered by public employees, and home-support services are contracted out to for-profit and not-for-profit agencies. In Nova Scotia and Manitoba, streamlining (case management and referral) functions are provided by public employees; professional services are provided by public employees or contracted out; and home-support services are contracted out to for-profit and not-for-profit agencies. Lastly, in Ontario, public employees provide case management and referral functions and professional and home-support services are contracted out to for-profit and not-for-profit agencies. In most provinces, home care programs are integrated with other health sectors through regional or local authorities, in others (e.g., Ontario), they stand alone.

Home care programs vary widely from province to province across Canada in how they are funded, the amount of funding devoted to them, who is eligible for their services, the amounts of services clients can receive, and who delivers them.

WHO USES HOME CARE?

The elderly and women are the main users of home care. In the absence of national data, Figure 5–1 shows the age-gender distribution of home care clients in Ontario. The majority of users were women (60.1 percent). Of the male home care clients, 50 percent were over the age of 65, whereas 65 percent of female home care clients were over 65.

Figure 5–2 shows the utilization rate (i.e., the number of home care clients per 1,000 population). While Figure 5–1 showed that

FIGURE 5 - 1

Age-Gender Distribution of Home Care Clients in Ontario, FY95

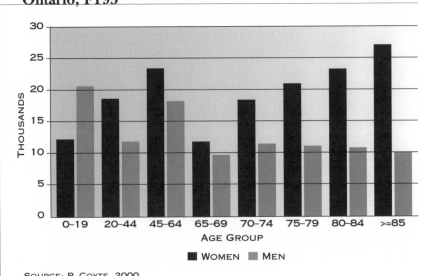

SOURCE: P. COYTE, 2000

FIGURE 5-2

Home Care Utilization Rates by Age and Gender in Ontario, FY95

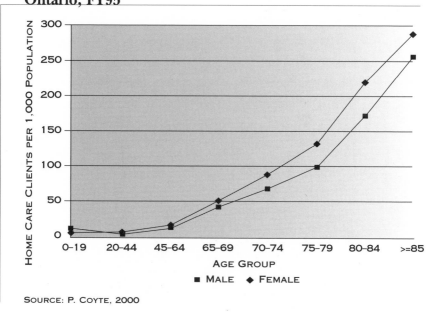

SOURCE: P. COYTE, 2000

the number of clients under the age of 65 is large, Figure 5–2 shows that, as a proportion of their age group, the utilization rate of those under 65 represent less than 2 percent compared to persons over the age of 65. Moreover, the utilization rate of women is more than 20 percent higher than that of men.

Figure 5–3 shows the intensity of home care utilization (i.e., the number of home care services or total cost of services for each home care client) by both age and gender. Not surprisingly, the intensity of home care use is higher for older people than younger people and higher for women than for men (except in the 20 to 44 age group). The impact of receiving care in the home is also felt more by women than by men. When in hospital, patients receive care and medication from hospital staff; their meals are prepared for them, their rooms are cleaned and they are helped with bathing. When they go home from hospital, or if they are elderly and are avoiding institutionalization, they may still need these services, but there is no guarantee that they will be provided by government. As

FIGURE 5 - 3

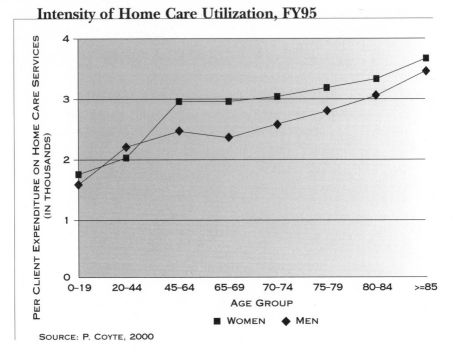

Intensity of Home Care Utilization, FY95

SOURCE: P. COYTE, 2000

a result, home care clients must rely in whole or in part on family and friends, the so-called "informal caregivers." While women are more often home care clients, they are also more often informal caregivers. Women are often in the position of both looking after children and their elderly parents. With more and more women in the workplace, the emotional and financial squeeze felt by women can be overwhelming.

GROWTH OF HOME CARE FUNDING AND PROVINCIAL VARIATION

There has been a dramatic growth in public home care expenditures in Canada in the last twenty-five years—from $62 million in 1975 to $2.1 billion in 1997 (see Figure 5–4). Moreover, since 1992 home care spending has grown at a rate four times greater than other health spending. However, these figures hide the fact that public home care spending still represents only 4 percent of total health care spending by the federal and provincial governments.

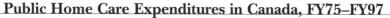

FIGURE 5-4

Public Home Care Expenditures in Canada, FY75–FY97

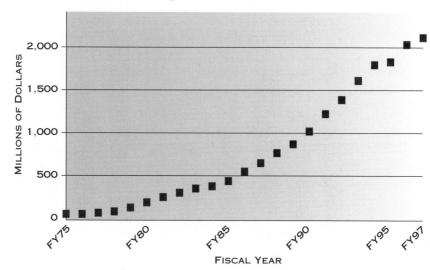

SOURCE: POLICY AND CONSULTATION BRANCH, HEALTH CANADA, MARCH 1998.
WWW.HC-SC.GC.CA/DATAPCB/DATAHESA/HOMECARE/HOMECARE. HTM, 1999.

The amount each province spends on home care also varies considerably even after adjusting for demographic differences between the regions. For example, in 1997 New Brunswick, followed by Newfoundland, Ontario, and Manitoba, spent more per person on home care than any other province, and the province that spent the most public money per person (New Brunswick) spent almost three times as much as the provinces that spent the least, PEI and Quebec (see Figure 5–5).

There are a number of factors that can account for the differences in home care spending across the country. To begin with, provinces differ in how much they can spend on health care in general, and so have different capabilities for allocating resources to the different sectors of health care. There is variation across the provinces in how much they use the home as a setting for care. Some regions make heavier use of community clinics, geriatric day-care centres, and so on. There is variation in the age-gender composition of the populations in each province. Each region is also at a different stage of health restructuring and therefore, differs in its emphasis on shifting care away from hospitals.

FIGURE 5-5

Public Home Care Expenditures Per Capita, FY97

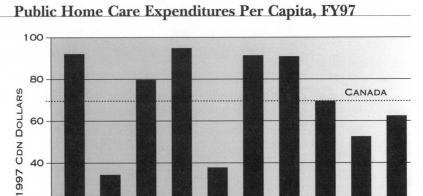

SOURCE: HEALTH CANADA, 1999

Nevertheless, this variation raises concerns as to whether all Canadians, regardless of where they live, have equal access to home care services in terms of the range and number of services, whether they are receiving the appropriate treatment, and the amount they must pay out-of-pocket. All these issues point to the need for national standards in this sector of care.

PASSIVE PRIVATIZATION: CHANGING SITES OF CARE AND CHANGING PATTERNS OF COSTS

As we stated earlier, both physicians' and hospital care in Canada fall under the Canada Health Act.[5] The five principles of universality, comprehensiveness, accessibility, portability, and public administration place conditions on federal transfers to the provinces and restrict the role that the private sector may play in financing health care. While Canada has a publicly *financed* health care system, it has a largely private, not-for-profit *delivery* system for medically necessary services.

Since home care services fall outside the CHA, they are, therefore, not protected by its five principles and do not have to be publicly funded—although, in fact, Ontario used to fund professional home care services before the 1990s through the Ontario Health Insurance Plan (OHIP) budget that pays for physicians' services, as long as the care was medically necessary. However, when it was reforming long-term care services, the NDP government took the home care budget out of the Ontario Health Insurance Plan budget and moved it to its own capped budget. The current Progressive Conservative government introduced stricter eligibility criteria and maximum levels of service per individual. As a result, care is fully funded when provided, but is not necessarily provided when needed. This becomes particularly important when we consider the changing nature of the home care population.

Traditionally, these services were provided to the elderly or to people with functional disabilities in order to allow them to live independently within the community. As more and more acute care (care covered under the CHA) for the general population has shifted from hospitals to the community, its provision no longer needs to conform to the five principles of the Canada Health Act. In fact, as acute care services move into the community, provincial governments that were formerly required to publically fund certain services are no longer under any legal obligation to do so. Despite governments' commitment to reallocate the funding that was freed up by the downsizing of hospitals to home care programs, this is not happening as quickly as the increase in need for services in the home.[6]

Provincial governments in Canada are able to take advantage of the fact that some health care services are being redefined as care that no longer falls under the funding requirements of the CHA. They can cut health care costs by moving services into these extra-CHA health sectors or by setting service maximums, as Ontario did. In this way, changing the site of care to the home means that there are no longer any national standards—or, of course, any penalties for breaches of standards—applied to such care. That loophole is allowing governments to erode the fabric of medicare to reduce their costs. Meanwhile, the financial burden on patients and their families is increasing, as they either have to pay directly for professional care or family members have to stay home from work to provide it themselves.

GROWTH IN PRIVATE SPENDING

As we noted in Chapter 2, private spending on health care has increased. It has been estimated that approximately 20 percent of the increase can be attributed to the fact that more services are available, and at higher costs, in the areas of health care that were always privately funded (active privatization). But about 80 percent of the increase is estimated to be due to what is called *passive privatization*, that is, governments no longer paying for services that were until recently publicly financed: services that have been delisted from the provincial medicare schedules and acute care services formerly available only in hospitals that are now being provided at home.

Not much is known about the amount of money Canadians spend privately on home care. The information that is available comes from a number of surveys. One recent survey indicated that 25 percent of home care clients say they pay an average of $407 per month for home care and $138 on prescription drugs.[7][8] Patients who were recently sent home from hospital spent approximately $200 per week on home care services. Other surveys by home care provider organizations have found that about 24.5 percent of the cost of nursing services and 59.3 percent of the cost of home support services are paid for directly by clients, with an average weekly out-of-pocket expenditure of $283.[9]

Although figures are not available, Peter Coyte of the Home Care Evaluation and Research Centre at the University of Toronto has estimated that in 1997 private payment for home care services was probably more than $500 million, and total spending on home care, public and private, was $2.62 billion. Private home care spending represents about 19.1 percent of total spending on home care. If this trend continues, we can expect home care to cost Canada, in total public and private spending, $3.4 billion in 2000–01.[10] However, this is not to imply that home care spending is out of control. Recall from Chapter 2 that Canada's total health care spending is now approaching $90 billion; $3.4 billion represents less than 4 percent of that total.

As we indicated earlier, the Canadian population is growing and aging; the proportion of Canadians over the age of 65 and over 80 is increasing. Based on the current uses and costs of home care, we can expect a 78.4 percent total increase in home care expenditures between 1999 and 2026 due to these demographic changes. How this will be paid for (i.e., publicly or privately) is an important reform decision that remains to be made.

THE NEED FOR EVIDENCE

The home care sector and its associated services are expanding very quickly, but we do not have enough information about costs, spending patterns, and utilization. Nor have we researched the quality, safety, effectiveness, relative efficiency, and accessibility of these services. Without information about the costs and consequences of home care services, we run the risk of making policy decisions that increase costs and erode health outcomes.[11] This risk is particularly evident in the growth of competitive and for-profit private home care insurance arrangements.

There are three assumptions that seem to be guiding the expansion of home care and the shifting of the site of non-hospital care to the home. The first assumption is that Canadians *want* to be responsible for health care delivery at home, and that people's family and support circumstances will allow them to stay at home to do so. However, staying at home usually involves a commitment from family members or friends, usually women, and we are already hearing of the burdens felt by women who are looking after both young children and elderly parents. Moreover, the fact that unprecedented numbers of women entered the work force over the last decades of the twentieth century means that we cannot safely assume that they will be a ready supply of informal caregiving, or that they can do so without substantial economic hardship.

Second, it is assumed that the home allows for safe and effective care to be provided. This assumption, too, is doubtful. Homes were never designed to be hospitals. It is true that increasingly complex conditions are now capable of being treated at home, and many treatments are more technically sophisticated, but we need to know whether the home is a safe site for acute or long-term care, and whether informal caregivers (such as friends and family members) can cope safely with what is being required of them.

Lastly, it is assumed that equal or better care at a lower cost will be the outcome of shifting care to the home. We are beginning to see the results of some research into this question, but much more is needed. For example, studies have found no evidence that light (preventive) levels of home care keep seniors alive longer or help them live independently for a longer period of time than seniors not receiving those services. In fact, the findings of a recent study by the Health Services Utilization and Research Commission contradict the assumption that home care is better and costs less. After adjusting for health status and use of other services, Saskatchewan seniors receiving preventive home care were 50 percent *more likely* to lose their independence, or die than those not receiving these services. In addition, the average total health service costs for preventive home care recipients were about triple the average costs for recipients of nursing homes or hospital care. On the other hand, residents of seniors' housing were 63 percent less likely to lose their independence and 40 percent less likely to die than other Saskatchewan seniors, while incurring about the same total health service costs as non-residents.[12] The results of this study suggests that better health outcomes, extended independence and lower costs are more likely to be achieved through seniors' housing than through preventive home care. This recent study, along with reviews of the international literature and work conducted for Ontario's Health Services Restructuring Commission,[13, 14, 15] provide a fairly extensive overview of the research available in the area; none of those sources found much compelling evidence to document the assertion that cheaper and more effective care is closer to home.[16, 17, 18]

A more recent study from British Columbia, by contrast, provides strong evidence for the cost and prevention effectiveness of social services.[19] In 1994 the British Columbia government instituted a policy of cutting services such as housekeeping to clients with minimal home care needs. While some regions in the province implemented this policy, others did not, creating a large-scale unplanned natural experiment. Comparison of the use of services and outcomes of those seniors who continued to receive homemaking services with those who were denied these services showed no difference between the groups in the first year after the cuts. However, the costs of care for those whose homemaking services had been cut increased substantially above the other group. In the third year, the annual costs per person for all health services for those who still received homemaking services averaged $7,808 compared with $11,903 for those who were denied the service. Three years after the cuts there was also a difference in outcomes. Seventeen percent of those whose services were cut entered long-term care institutions compared to 7 percent who continued to receive homemaking services. Twenty-two percent in the former group had died three years after the cut compared with 15 percent in the latter group. The authors conclude that these cheaper social services are not only cheaper, but also appear to help maintain the functioning of elderly persons and prevent their deterioration.

NATIONAL STANDARDS FOR HOME CARE

Publicly insured medically necessary care is under threat of being de-insured as it moves closer to home. This is changing the contours of medicare as we know it and debases the idea of public insurance for medically required services. With capped budgets in home care, acute care clients are being given priority for dwindling funded services and accessibility of care is undermined; waiting lists are becoming common. Traditional clients of home care—the elderly and people with chronic disabilities—have to wait longer for care, pay privately, or do without.

Home care has always been partially publicly funded. However, with the aging of the population and the shifting site of care, the financial, emotional, and time burdens on patients and their families and friends are increasing. As Figure 5–5 indicates very clearly, the public spending picture on home care varies considerably from province to province (by a factor of three). Canadians are certainly not getting equal access to home care. While many champion home care as the new frontier, it is more than just a new way of providing care. It may quickly become *the* way in which the majority of care is provided.

The shifting site of care, the passive privatization of health costs through home care, and the provincial variation in programs are all warning signals of the urgent need for Canada to establish a national standard for home care. Without such a standard Canadians will not be able to count on having the universal, accessible, comprehensive, portable, and publicly administered care that they want and expect.

We have a number of options available to us to create a pan-Canadian standard for home care. We can extend the five principles of the Canada Health Act by including home care under the category of insured services, so that there would be a common base of services (a floor of covered services) available and accessible to all Canadians on the same conditions no matter where they reside in Canada. At the same time, we would need to build in incentives to ensure that all provinces honour the standards and are held accountable for doing so.

Another option would be to develop a separate agreement between the federal government and the provinces through, for example, the Social Union Framework Agreement adopted by the first ministers in late 1997. The agreement would be enforced through conditional federal funding specifically targeted for home care services, such that provinces would not be permitted to use these funds in any other way. In order to receive these new funds, provinces would need to provide a common base of home care services under uniform eligibility criteria.

A third option would be to develop a separate social insurance program for home care as both Germany and Japan have recently done. The German national insurance program for home care and residential services is financed through a mandatory tax on salary (shared between employers and employees) and premiums paid by retirees and their pension funds. The program is for people with a mental or physical condition that results in a need for assistance in the activities of daily living and is expected to last at least six months. Benefits are fixed by the assessed level of disability. Clients can opt for the services or cash assistance. Although there is no monitoring of how the cash is spent, those who opt for the cash are monitored to ensure that adequate care is being provided. So far, the German program has been operating at less than budgeted projections. While the separate fund ensures that acute care services do not encroach on long-term-care budgets, it does maintain certain rigidities between care sectors. [20, 21]

In 2000 Japan also instituted a program of public, mandatory long-term-care insurance. There are two categories of insured persons:

1) those between the ages of 40 and 64; and 2) those aged 65 and over. The state (at national, provincial, and municipal levels) provides 50 percent of the program funding; persons over 65 provide 17 percent of the program funding through premiums; and those between the ages of 40 and 64 contribute 33 percent of the funding through premiums. Eligible clients are assessed in two stages, using a standardized assessment tool. Benefits are determined according to the assessed level of disability. There is a 10 percent service cost, which is controversial in Japan.[22, 23, 24]

These options are attempts to fund a national program of home care that ensures that benefits are distributed according to need and paid for according to means. However, setting national standards for home care in Canada, as the National Forum on Health[25] recommended, will not be easy. Provinces are at different stages of readiness and willingness to accept change and adopt common standards. Difficult decisions as to what services should be publicly funded will have to be made no matter what option we adopt. Some advocate covering only services that are thought to be "medically necessary" or that would have been previously provided either by a physician or in a hospital. Others call for the coverage of some social services, arguing that not only are these services key in the prevention of deteriorating health, which can lead to greater costs, but that they are also necessary for health services to be effective.

All of these matters, however, must be referred back to one fundamental question: what is the responsibility of government versus the individual in the provision and maintenance of people's health? Should the government pay for someone to clean your house or provide you with meals, things that a lot of Canadians already pay for when they are well and do not consider "health services"? Should people take full financial and other responsibility for their aging parents and ailing family members as they did in the past, before universal health care was established? We must tackle these difficult questions directly. Doing nothing will not preserve the status quo. Health care is changing whether or not the public wants it to. The question is whether we want to control and determine change or have change overtake us unprepared. Home care is a significant and growing part of health care. Thirty years ago, Canadians decided that national standards for medically necessary services were desirable and morally the right thing to do. The nature and site of care has changed, but the principles that we adopted under the Canada Health Act—that care should be *comprehensive, accessible, universal, portable,* and *publicly administered*—may well have application here. Unless we move quickly to establish some form of national standard in home care, it will continue to be the zone of passive privatization and gross inequities from province to province. This is simply not good enough!

The Future: Rigid, Resilient, or Retail Reform Choices

GREEN POULTICE OR FEDERAL INVESTMENT?

In the early 1990s difficult decisions had to be made to reduce health expenditures in Canada. These decisions arose as a natural consequence of shrinking government revenues and debt growth. Notwithstanding the bruising of our citizens' trust in our system that occurred at that time, we have made significant and needed adjustment in the numbers of hospitals and total beds available, and begun the dramatic shift of care to the community. We have also managed to rein in our debt growth and the higher levels of government in Canada have all moved to balance their books.

At the First Ministers' meeting in September 2000, the government of Canada began to plan reinvestment in health care as the first step towards restoring confidence in our shaken system. This was indeed welcome news and an indication that our fiscal house is in better shape. It is a positive change in federal action on health care, with important new ideas and investments in information infrastructure and child health, among other things. But in the absence of any plans to expand the range of services covered, this new spending is not sufficient by any means nor does the transfer deal with fiscal shocks and business cycle effects on government spending. Indeed, as the economy slowed in 2001, provincial and federal governments were once again looking at ways to constrain health care costs.

As we have noted, home care requires some form of national standard to ensure comparable access for all Canadians to a comparable range of services. As it stands right now, a threefold variation exists from province to province in the public funding of home care. Canadians are not entitled to the same level of publicly funded home care from one province to another. This was presumably quite adequate in the era when hospital care was the norm. However, in a time when more and more care is being provided in the home and the community, the passive privatization of necessary care will not serve the citizens of Canada well in the coming years. Some federal-provincial agreement must be reached on standards for home care or we will slowly begin to abandon the subsidy principle of medicare, the simplicity of our payment arrangements, and the cost control associated with public payment.

As stated in Chapter 5, the setting of national standards can be accomplished in a number of ways. The Canada Health Act could be extended by an intergovernmental agreement to include home care services or a new federal act could be created to cover home care for all Canadians. However, in the absence of a national standard in home care, provincial variation in the public financing of home care is likely to diverge even more, creating a nation of haves and have-nots in the new and emerging area of community health services. The important principles of solidarity behind the Canada Health Act can either be extended in some way to home care services, in recognition of the new realities of health care, or they can remain as they are now, limited to the smaller core of hospital and medical services leaving every citizen and every province to their own devices for home care.

To those who would say that home care is a private financing responsibility and should not be brought into the domain of publicly financed care, we reply that this view ignores the realities of modern health care delivery. Our health care system is based, among other things, on the belief that low-income families should not be bankrupted by having to pay in advance for an emergency heart attack. Should we then stand by as a community and allow the same families to be bankrupted by expensive home care following shorter and more complex cardiovascular surgery, which requires extensive home care for the recovery period? Should we allow them to be bankrupted by extensive home care costs for congestive heart failure in the elderly or for the care of a medically fragile child with a congenital heart defect?

A Canadian standard can be achieved most effectively through setting conditions on the transfer of federal money. To date there have been no new conditions to compel any change in the scope of health care coverage in Canada, nor has there been any federal-provincial framework agreement that establishes the base standard within a specific context, such as the social union framework. In either case, the role of the federal government is crucial to ensure a trans-Canada highway in health care.

In the case of waiting lists, nothing short of an all-out assault across the jurisdictions in Canada is required. A more effective management of the delivery and allocation processes is required to reduce wait lists and times. The simple addition of new money will not solve the problem and may, indeed, be counter-productive in some instances.

Although we have not addressed *all* health reform priorities in this book, at least two other areas are also in urgent need of reform: pharmaceuticals and primary care. In the case of pharmaceuticals, as with home care, no base of public insurance is currently specified across Canada. Major variations exist. While drug prices in Canada are the fastest-growing area of public expenditure, Canadians still pay less than 90 percent of the median international world price for drugs, generating repeated calls for U.S. citizens to be able to purchase drugs directly from Canadian sources.[1] There has been some limited control of pharmaceutical cost growth through the Patented Medicine Prices Review Board (www.pmprb-cepmb.gc.ca), a weak price-regulation mechanism introduced as a consequence of NAFTA. Nevertheless, greater efficiencies are still possible through a single-payer, publicly financed plan. The federal government is once again extremely well positioned to coordinate the insurance function for pharmaceutical services in this country, should they wish to take it on. However, the government of Canada appears to have little appetite for launching the kind of complex checkerboard program that will be necessary to build a national pharmaceutical program, even though the National Forum on Health, appointed by the federal government, recommended such a program.

In the area of primary care reform, the dimensions requiring change are *delivery* and *allocation* of resources, not financing. Many

Canadian hospitals and health care organizations, particularly in academic centres, are already moving towards some form of alternative payment scheme or salary-based arrangement for physicians. The parallel change of payment arrangements for most general and family practice physicians is necessary for the reform of primary care. With such reform, many physicians, nurse practitioners, and other health providers can work together under a salary arrangement, to deliver appropriate and more seamless care. However, despite the weight of evidence and significant support from individual physicians for this type of reform, there is entrenched resistance from some sectors of organized medicine because of their attachment to fee-for-service medicare and the desire of some medical associations to be the sole bargaining agents for doctors. As we noted earlier, the crowding of emergency rooms has less to do with the funding of hospital ER facilities and far more to do with primary care reform and the integration of staged community and home care into the continuum of covered services.

Despite these pressing reform imperatives, the way in which Canada *finances* health care—a single-payer publicly financed mechanism—is in our view very sound. Reform of the key areas mentioned above can all be achieved within this financing framework without bankrupting us. Our financing mechanism should be cherished as one that reflects and supports our civic values. However, as discussed, because of international trade agreements the Canadian health care system faces possible challenges from transnational for-profit interests, that threaten this unique aspect of our system. The passive and active movement of publicly insured services into areas dominated by both public and private financing and delivery, such as home care and pharmaceuticals, make them susceptible to off-shore interests.[2, 3, 4, 5] Once these interests have a foothold in Canada, such private stakes will not only be hard to reverse but may well lead to a weak national standard in health care.

Home care, waiting lists, pharmaceutical coverage, and primary care are critical areas requiring reform in Canada. The maintenance of *confidence* in our health care system and the preservation of an efficient single-payer public financing mechanism depends on action on these fronts. As we have seen, all developed countries are facing challenges in sustaining public confidence and Canada is no exception. In this book, we have chosen to focus on waiting lists and home care because we believe Canada has achieved a political consensus for change in these areas. What is required is the creation of some federal political will motivated by public action to move the agenda forward.

Despite a lack of federal action, some provinces are moving ahead. Quebec is not inactive. It has already made important moves in many social policy areas in advance of the rest of Canada. Notwithstanding its own imperfections, Quebec recently introduced a payroll-financed pharmacare plan to cover its citizens. In addition, the recent Clair Commission Report in Quebec also touched on primary care reform, suggesting the development of group practices among physicians and nurses. Such practices would serve a roster of 1,000 to 1,800 patients out of their own clinics or in association with Quebec's well-established community health and social service centres (CLSCs).

Perhaps most provocative, the Clair Commission Report has recommended the creation of a *new public fund* to begin to deal with growing home care costs. This new social insurance fund would presumably require statutory payroll contributions to cover "loss of autonomy," i.e., long-term care for the elderly and the chronically ill.[6] This is an interesting proposal in view of the developments in such dedicated social insurance funds in Germany and Japan noted in Chapter 5. Payroll-financed group insurance programs, such as the loss-of-autonomy fund suggested by Clair, are more common in European approaches to health insurance and require careful regulatory surveillance to prevent cost shifting and risk shifting of more expensive care.

The Clair Commission Report also called for a greater role for private partnership, especially to accelerate the use of technology. Quebec, which has always been an innovator in social policy, appears ready to make some changes to its own public system to reform home care, long-term care, pharmacare, and primary care.

The homeland of medicare in Canada, Saskatchewan, has also received some recent guidance for its reform plan from the Fyke Commission.[7] The recommendations included the harsh medicine of slimming down hospitals to increase the quality of high-volume procedures, the creation of larger regions, and the creation of a provincial quality council. The Fyke Commission also recommended bold moves in the direction of primary care reform, including the integration of physician services in the regional budget envelopes and the creation of primary care networks. If the recommendation is acted upon, this step towards integrating physician services in regional budgets will be the first of its kind in Canada to allow the regional health authority to organize its own approaches to physicians' services. These rich provincial proposals for change are important examples of reform issues to be dealt with by the Romanow Federal Commission on the Future of Health Care in Canada.

THREE REFORM FUTURES

In Tables 6–1, and 6–2, we have set out three simplified sketches of possible reform scenarios for Canada and compared how they would perform in relation to the key features of our system (Table 6–1) as sketched early on in Chapter 1. We also compare how they are likely to affect financing and coverage within the Canadian system (Table 6–2).

The *Rigid* scenario involves muddling along more or less as we have been. This is the continuation of a world in which the essential services covered in a national health plan include doctors and hospital services with at least some drugs and some home care services available to most Canadians. Conditions attached to federal transfers exert some discipline on the provinces, but the shifting nature of the coverage for health care and the susceptibility of the system to fiscal shocks (such as occurred in the early 1990s) render the system less responsive than it might be. Costs are continuously and passively shifted to the private purses of individuals and employers.

In the *Resilient* future, new federal transfer conditions are imposed on the provinces to extend a base of flexible public coverage to home and community care and pharmaceuticals. This will certainly involve federal-provincial negotiation and will almost certainly require an agreement to allow fully formed provincial plans that meet the federal standard to qualify for federal transfers (as the Quebec pension plan meets the basic objectives of the Canada Pension Plan). This idea, called asymmetric federalism, is one way of

TABLE 6-1
The Survival of Desirable Elements in Three Reform Futures

	SUBSIDY FEATURES	SIMPLICITY	GROWTH OF COSTS		
			PUBLIC	PRIVATE	TOTAL SPENDING (PUBLIC PLUS PRIVATE)
RIGID FUTURE	Physicians' services, hospital services, and some public services are provided based on need and funded according to income Other services involve supplementary insurance and out of pocket costs	One payer for most medically necessary services across Canada Other services involve co-insurance and out-of-pocket with significant provincial variation	Slow growth of public costs, continued shift to more expensive private coverage as community care grows		
			+	++	+
RESILIENT FUTURE	Key subsidy and transfer features of existing system expanded to new sites of care	National standard for broader range of services; reduced overhead and complexity; high level of transparency	Growth of public costs with broader scope of coverage; slow growth of private costs; overall growth of costs moderated by largely single payer		
			++	+	+
RETAIL FUTURE	Support for comprehensive public coverage wanes as solidarity towards financing mechanism wanes. Wealthier Canadians want to opt out of public payment.	Two levels of regulation required with significant provincial variation Multipayer environment and competitive plans increase complexity and reduce transparency	Modest crowding out (reduction) of public spending as a consequence of private spending growth; private costs grow more rapidly in multipayer environment; total costs go up significantly.		
			+	++	++

TABLE 6-2
Implications for Public Finance and Citizenship in Three Reform Futures

	FEDERAL FINANCING CONDITIONS	HOW SERVICES ARE FUNDED	CITIZENSHIP MODEL
RIGID FUTURE	Status Quo	Doctors and hospitals publicly covered Other health services cost shared with firms and individuals	Most medically necessary services as of right for citizens Variation in public home care and pharmaceutical services exist from province to province
RESILIENT FUTURE	Strengthened federal cash transfer conditions to accommodate technological change and changing sites of care; specified minimum standards for home, community, and pharmaceuticals by provinces (provincial asymmetry in programs allowed)	Public coverage extended from doctors and hospitals to include a flexible base of coverage for home, community care, and pharmaceuticals	All medically necessary services as of right for citizens regardless of site of care Common national standards of service for essential health services in all provinces in Canada
RETAIL FUTURE	Reduction of federal conditions to allow a "second tier" of private care, fully financed privately, as in the U.K., while ensuring a minimum base of public services	Two standards of coverage: first class and coach Private tier to be defined by market place (with regulation) Minimum public base of coverage	Basic medical/catastrophic services as of right for citizens Ability to pay moves you to the front of the line Checkerboard federalism emerges with quite different provincial plans, coverage, and interprovincial payment restrictions

trying to get comparable levels of public service at comparable levels of taxation without imposing federal cookie-cutters on the provinces' programs.

The *Retail* scenario is one in which consumer "freedom" trumps the freedoms, entitlements, and responsibilities of citizenship. Private financing as a solution succeeds as a meme, which replicates itself so relentlessly that it is adopted everywhere as the putative solution regardless of the international and Canadian evidence. It lets the genie of second-tier health care out of the bottle, and a common standard of service for all Canadians never returns.

In order to achieve this future, federal spending conditions must be altered and limited to a base of medically necessary services, while allowing for those with means to purchase private insurance to cut to the front of the line. Since health care is a provincial jurisdiction, provinces may choose (as they do now) to prohibit such options in their own jurisdictions (as we noted in Chapter 3), but the current federal financial restriction on supplementary payments for medically necessary services would be relaxed, allowing the possibility for two tiers of service to emerge in some provinces. In this scenario, it is most likely that *public* spending levels would actually decline modestly. A recent careful comparison of spending across OECD countries showed that increases in private spending on health care over time are associated with declines in public spending. A 10 percent increase in overall private spending will only be associated with 1 to 3 percent decline in public spending.[8] In other words, this increase in private spending is not offset by an equivalent decrease in public spending.

We have argued that the retail scenario would result in a significant increase in overall costs, while eliminating the simplicity and equity features of the Canadian system that we outlined at the beginning of Chapter 1. There is likely to be modest reduction in "coach" or public-class services and significant inflation in "first-class" or the private-tier services.

The health care system we have built in this country has been widely admired and reported upon. The Canada Health Act has served the Canadian public well. Canadians in the most part have received medically necessary care without being in jeopardy of financial risk. However, health care has changed significantly since the Canada Health Act was framed. The changing nature and site of care and the outdated coverage of the Canada Health Act are endangering the principles of equitable access to comprehensive care—care that Canadians have come to expect. In our fear of losing what we have, we have placed the Canada Health Act on a pedestal and held up our crossed fingers against the devils who wish to dismantle it. However, unlike some biblical edict, the Canada Health Act is not written in stone. In our view, we need a reform future that allows us to move from rigidity to resilience. Our legal framework for health care must be revitalized and embody a mechanism for the adaptation of public coverage to changing sites of care. Public coverage for necessary care must be flexible enough to ensure that Canadians are protected and receive the care they need no matter how or where that care is provided.

The time for reform is now. Change is overdue. Most health care analysts and decision makers know what needs to be done and the best ways of achieving it. What is required is action to create informed public discussion and propel political leadership. The leadership of our professional organizations, the leadership of the various managers and policy actors in our system, and patient coalitions must find some common voice. This is how Canadians got national health insurance to begin with. We must move to the next logical step in extending coverage for home and community care.

Because health care is a provincial jurisdiction, the provinces are the major parties in organizing and providing care for its citizens. This arrangement allows each province to express its local preferences to some degree. However, if Canada is to be more than just a collection of provinces, we must imbue our health care with uniquely Canadian values. The role of the federal government in the protection of these values, in our view, remains essential. It is the federal government that is best situated to ensure national standards, ideals, and integrity, even if some provinces are less than enthusiastic about any form of federal involvement. In an era of increasing incursion from off-shore corporations and pressure for economic "harmonization" from international trade agreements, unchecked provincial action in traded areas of health care can jeopardize these programs. The federal government, as the sole signatory to international trade agreements, must be the guardian of our social programs to ensure that Canadians continue to decide the kind of country they wish to live in.

It remains to be seen whether the government of Canada and the provincial governments can move beyond the rhetoric of jurisdictional and regional posturing disputes. Throwing money at our health care problems is simply an attempt to apply the "green poultice" to a set of problems that require political resolve, not only money. An unconditional influx of new federal transfer money in the fall of 2000, although welcome, fell far short of the action necessary to modernize the base of public health care coverage in this country.

The provinces have struggled with their own processes of reform, without much steering from the federal government. However, a concerted and unified effort by citizen groups, employer organizations, and both levels of government is required if we are to motivate our federal government to do the right thing in this most Canadian of policy arenas.

In a fundamental way, we Canadians must decide if we are to carve out a truly Canadian future for our health care system, consistent with our national character and unique constitutional values. For almost half a century these values have allowed us to ensure that those regions with means lend tax and transfer support for public services to those regions and fellow Canadians of lesser means. The public pooling of health spending in Canada has served our citizens well and appears to be at least one factor in our overall better health in comparison to our American cousins. It would be a mistake to shrug off these values as anachronisms in a time when consumerism trumps citizenship. A proper assessment of which health reform futures do more good than harm will require some careful national mirror-gazing on what we value as a nation. Let's hope we take each other into consideration.

E N D N O T E S

PREFACE ➤

1 Background papers prepared for the Dialogue on Health Reform from which material for this book is largely and shamelessly drawn are available in full, free of charge, from the University of Toronto at www.utoronto.ca/hpme/dhr/4. html. A number of these papers have since been revised as free-standing papers. These papers include:

"Getting What We Pay For: Myths and Realities about Financing Canada's Health Care System." Raisa B. Deber, Department of Health Policy, Management and Evaluation, University of Toronto, May 29, 2000.

"Waiting for Medical Services in Ontario: Clarifying the Issues in a Period of Health Reform." Sam Shortt, Director, Queen's University Health Policy Group, May 29, 2000.

"Waiting for Health Care in Canada: Problems and Prospects." Morris Barer, Director UBC Centre for Health Services and Policy Research and Steven Lewis, Access Consulting, Saskatoon, June 15, 2000.

"Home Care in Canada: Passing the Buck." Peter Coyte, Dept. of Health Policy, Management and Evaluation, University of Toronto, June 16, 2000.

"Care in the Home: Public Responsibility—Private Roles?" Malcolm Anderson, and Karen Parent, Dept. of Rehabilitation Medicine, Queen's University, August 21, 2000.

"Legal Constraints on Privately-Financed Health Care in Canada: A Review of the Ten Provinces." Colleen Flood, and Tom Archibald, candidate, Faculty of Law, University of Toronto, September 4, 2000.

"The National Leadership Roundtable on Health Reform." Dialogue on Health Reform, Dept. of Health Policy, Management and Evaluation, University of Toronto. Report prepared by Dr. Alina Gildner.

CHAPTER 1 ➤ Declining Public Confidence in Canada's Health Care System

1 The Dialogue on Health Reform was created in 1999, with support from the Atkinson Foundation, in order to stimulate a balanced discussion of the problems facing the Canadian health care system, act as a counterbalance to more extreme and misinformed solutions, and

advocate for reform based on evidence. Members of the Dialogue agree on the soundness of the financing mechanisms in the Canadian health care system. The Dialogue has undertaken a number of activities to further a balanced discourse. It commissioned several background papers from experts in health care on a number of issues that have been hot spots of misinformation. In June of 2000, the Dialogue hosted a National Leadership Roundtable on Health Reform that brought together thinkers from diverse fields (academics, business people, care providers, consumers, former politicians, and American health care experts). Background on the Dialogue, its steering committee, membership, topical papers, and public commentary can be found on the Dialogue web site: http://www.utoronto.ca/hpme/dhr.

2   Angus Reid Group, National Poll # 53 (1999).

3   F.P.T. Advisory Group on Population Health, *Toward a Healthy Future*, Second Report on the Health of Canadians (Ottawa: Ministry of Public Works and Government Services, 1999). While we were for many years number 1 on the U.N. Human Development Index, we rank poorly on the Human Poverty Index. See United Nations Development Report, 1998, a factor that is associated with our recent fall to the number 3 position.

4   For a most complete discussion of different notions of freedom, see Isaiah Berlin, "Two Views of Liberty," in M. Sandel, ed., *Liberalism and Its Critics* (New York: New York University Press, 1984).

5   T. Sullivan and C. Mustard, "Canada: More State, More Market?" in John Davis, ed., *The Social Economics of Healthcare* (New York: Routledge, 2001).

6   N. A. Ross, M. C. Wolfson, J. R. Dunn, J. M. Berthelot, G. A. Kaplan, and J. W. Lynch, "Relation between Income Inequality and Mortality in Canada and in the United States: Cross Sectional Assessment Using Census Data and Vital Statistics," *British Medical Journal* 320 (2000): 898–902.

7   J. Frank and F. Mustard, "The Rise in the Health of Populations and Historical Change in Population Health," *Daedalus* 123(4) (1994): 1–21.

8   *Health Care in Canada*, (Ottawa: Canadian Institute for Health Information, 2001), 60–61.

9   Angus Reid, "Health Care in Canada" (February 2000).

10 Angus Reid (May 1999).

11 Ekos Research Associates Inc., "Canadian Values in Health Policy," presentation at the Centre for Health Economics and Policy Analysis Policy Conference (May 18, 2000).

12   Ekos Research, *Rethinking Government*, (December 1999).

13   Angus Reid (February 2000).

14   Ontario Hospital Association, *Hospital Report '99: A Balanced Scorecard for Ontario Acute Care Hospitals* (December 1999).

15   Canadian Institute for Health Information, *Health Care in Canada: A First Annual Report* (2000). Also S. Ships, R. Reid, H. Krueger, K. McGrail, B. Green, et al, "Hospital Downsizing and Trends in Health Care Use among Elderly People in British Columbia," *Canadian Medical Association Journal* 163(4) (2000): 397–401. Also N. Roos, "The Disconnect between the Data and the Headlines," *Canadian Medical Association Journal* 163(4) (2000): 411.

16   Ontario Hospital Association (1999).

17   K. Donelan, R. Blendon, C. Schoen, K. Davis, and K. Binns, " The Cost of Health System Change: Public Discontent in Five Nations," *Health Affairs* 18(3) (May/June 1999).

18   C. Schoen, K. Davis, C. DesRoches, K. Donelan, R. Blendon, and E. Strumpf, "Equity in Health Care across Five Nations: Summary Findings from an International Survey," *The Commonwealth Fund Issue Brief* (May 2000).

19   K. Davis, *Common Concerns: International Issues in Health Care System Reform*, The Commonwealth Fund, *Annual Report*: President's Message (1998).

20   G. F. Anderson, J. P. Poullier, "Health Spending, Access and Outcomes: Trends in Industrialized Countries," *Health Affairs* 18(3) (May/June, 1999).

21   Ibid.

22   Ibid.

23   B. Starfield, *Primary Care: Balancing Health Needs, Services and Technology* (New York: Oxford University Press, 1998).

24   *World Health Report(2000)*.   http://www.who.int/whr/2000/an/report.htm.

25   L. Kohn, J. Corrigan, and M. Donaldson, eds., *To Err is Human: Building a Safer Health System* (Washington, DC: National Academy Press, 1999).

26   B. Starfield, "Is US Health Really the Best in the World?" Commentary, *Journal of the American Medical Association* 284(4) (2000): 483–85.

27   In addition to these problem areas, the mix, distribution, supply, and

compensation mechanisms for professionals remain areas of growing concern, although we will not be addressing these directly.

28 Ekos Research Associates Inc. (2000).

29 D. Price, A. Pollock, J. Shaoul, "How the World Trade Organisation Is Shaping Domestic Policies in Health Care," *Lancet* 354 (November 27, 1999): 1889–92.

30 B. Appleton, "International Agreements and National Health Plans: NAFTA," in D. Drache, and T. Sullivan, eds., *Health Reform, Public Success Private Failure,* (London: Routledge, 1999).

31 B. Appleton, "NAFTA Investment Chapter Implications of Alberta Bill 11," legal opinion to the Canadian Health Coalition, (April 10, 2000).

32 S. Shrybman, "A Legal Opinion concerning NAFTA Investment and Services Disciplines and Bill 11: Proposals by Alberta to Privatize the Delivery of Certain Health Services," legal opinion to the Canadian Union of Public Employees (March 2000).

33 C. Tuohy, *Accidental Logics: The Dynamics of Change in the Health Care Arena in the United States, Britain and Canada* (New York: Oxford University Press, 1999).

34 R. Evans, "Two Systems in Restraint: Contrasting Experiences with Cost Control in the 1990s," in D. M. Thomas, ed., *Canada and the United States: Differences that Count,* (Peterborough, Ontario: Broadview, 2000), 21–51.

35 T. Sullivan, M. Kerr, and S. Ibrahim, "Job Stress in Healthcare Workers: Highlights from the National Population Health Survey," *Hospital Quarterly* (Summer 1999). See also M. Koehoorn, and T. Sullivan, "The Health of Nursing Personnel: A Summary of Research Findings to Inform the Development of a National Survey in Canada," background paper prepared for the Office of Nursing Policy (2001).

36 C. Tuohy, *Accidental Logics: The Dynamics of Change in the Health Care Arena in the United States, Britain and Canada* (New York: Oxford University Press, 1999).

37 T. Marmor, "An American Diagnosis: If It Ain't Broke, Don't Fix It," opinion piece in the *Globe and Mail* (May 15, 2000). See also T. Marmor and K. Sullivan, "Canada's Burning! Media Myths About Universal Health Insurance," *The Washington Monthly* (July/August 2000): 15–20.

38 *More Money Would Put an End to Emergency Room Crunches,* Canadian Health Services Research Foundation Mythbusters Series #1 (2000).

See also V. Menec, "Seasonal Patterns of Winnipeg Hospital Use," Manitoba Centre for Health Policy and Evaluation.

CHAPTER 2 ➤ What Is Public and What Is Private?

1   Much of the material in this chapter is derived from or uses material from R. Deber, "Getting What We Pay For: Myths and Realities about Financing Canada's Health Care System," and C. Flood and T. Archibald, "Legal Constraints on Privately-Financed Health Care in Canada: A Review of the Ten Provinces," two reports prepared for the Dialogue on Health Reform (2000).

2   This does not necessarily mean it must be administered directly by a ministry of government. It could be administered through an agency, commission, or quasi-public insurer that is more or less private but regulated carefully by the government. This is effectively how most hospitals and regional authorities operate in Canada.

3   R. Evans "What Business Is It of Business," in D. Drache and T. Sullivan, *Public Success, Private Failure: Market Limits in Health Reform* (New York: Routledge, 1999).

4   S. Glied and M. Stabile, "Generation Vexed: Age-Cohort Differences in Employer Sponsored Health Insurance," *Health Affairs* 20(1) (2001): 184–91.

5   K. Grumbach and T. Bodenheimer, "Reins or Fences: Physicians' View of Cost Containment," *Health Affairs* 9(4) (1990): 120–26.

6   R. Evans and N. Roos, "What Is Right about the Canadian Health Care System," *Millbank Quarterly*, 77(3) (1999): 393-99.

7   National Forum on Health, *Canada Health Action: Building on the Legacy* (St. Foy, Quebec: Editions Multimondes, 1997).

CHAPTER 3 ➤ Memes and Myths

1   See R. Brodie, *Virus of the Mind: The New Science of the Meme* (Seattle: Integral Press, 1996).

2   Much of this chapter is taken from R. Deber, "Getting What We Pay For: Myths and Realities about Financing Canada's Health Care System," and C. Flood and T. Archibald, "Legal Constraints on Privately-Financed Health Care in Canada: A Review of the Ten Provinces," two reports prepared for the Dialogue on Health Reform (2000).

3   These are modified examples inspired by R. Deber (2000).

4   T. Sullivan, "New Life or Green Poultice?" review of the Commission on the NHS, *Canadian Medical Association Journal*, 163(10) (2000): 117–18.

5   W. Armstrong, "The Consumer Experience with Cataract Surgery and Private Clinics in Alberta: Canada's Canary in the Mine Shaft" (Alberta: The Consumer's Association of Canada, January 2000).

6   R. Wilson, opening remarks in *Access to Quality Health Care For All Canadians: Proceedings of the National Health Policy Summit*, Montebello, Canadian Medical Association (1996), 11.

7   This section draws heavily on C. Flood and T. Archibald, Legal Constraints on Privately-Financed Health Care in Canada."

8   S. Sheps, R. Reid, M. Barer, H. Krueger, K. McGrail, B. Green, R. Evans, and C. Hertzman, "Hospital Downsizing and Health Care Use among Elderly People in British Columbia," *Canadian Medical Association Journal*, 163(4) (2000): 397–401.

9   J. F. Fries, "Compression of Morbidity in the Elderly," *Vaccine*, 18(16) (2000): 1584–89.

10 R. Deber (2000).

11 R. Evans, M. Barer, and G. Stoddart, "Charging Peter to Pay Paul: Accounting for the Financial Effects of User Fees," Premier's Council on Health, Well Being & Social Justice (1994).

12 I. Peritz, "Fees Deter Quebec Sick from Getting Help," *Globe and Mail*, (Saturday, March 27, 1999).

CHAPTER 4 ➤ Canaries in the Mine: Waiting for Care

1   This chapter draws heavily from two papers prepared for the Dialogue on Health Reform (2000): S. E. D. Shortt, "Waiting for Medical Services in Ontario: Clarifying the Issues in a Period of Health Reform," and M. L. Barer, and S. Lewis, "Waiting for Health Care in Canada: Problems and Prospects."

2   S. Lewis, and C. Sanmartin, "Managing Waiting Lists to Achieve Distributive Justice," a working paper prepared for the Western Canada Wait List Project (2001).

3   Ironically, shipping cancer patients to the U.S. for treatment is a very expensive proposition, which is why solutions that build on improving local capacity to respond are preferable.

4   Paul McDonald, et al, "Waiting Lists and Waiting Times for Health Care in Canada: More Management! More Money?" http://www.hc-sc.gc.ca/iacb-dgiac/nhrdp/wlsum5.htm (1998)

5   "Waiting Your Turn," The Fraser Institute (2000).

6   *A Parallel Private System Would Reduce Waiting Times in the Public System,* Canadian Health Services Research Foundation Mythbusters Series No. 2.

7   J. I. Williams, H. Llewellyn-Thomas, R. Arshinoff, N. Young, C.D. Naylor, et al, "The Burden Waiting for Hip and Knee Replacements in Ontario." *Journal of Evaluation in Clinical Practice* 3 (1997): 59–68.

8   M. Rigge, "Quality of Life of Long Wait Orthopaedic Patients Before and After Admission: A Consumer Audit." *Quality in Health Care* 3 (1994): 159–63.

9   J. C. Hall, J. L. Hall, "The Quality of Life of Patients on a Waiting List for Transurethral Resection of the Prostate." *Journal of Quality in Clinical Practice* 16 (1996): 69–73.

10 T. Rector, S. Ormaza, S. Kubo, "Health Status of Heart Transplant Recipients versus Patients Awaiting Heart Transplantation: A Preliminary Evaluation of the SF–36 Questionnarie." *Journal of Heart and Lung Transplantation* 12 (1993): 983–86.

11 N. Lee, K. Claridge, G. Thompson, "Do We Require Initiatives to Reduce Outpatient Waiting Lists?" *Health Trends* 24 (1992): 30–33.

12 A. Freeland and J. Curley, "The Consequences of Delay in Tonsil Surgery." *Otolaryngology Clinics of North America* 20 (1987): 405–08.

13 M. Bishop, "The Dangers of a Long Urological Waiting List." *British Journal of Urology* 65 (1990): 433–40.

14 K. Hartford and L. L. Roos, "Does Waiting Time for Coronary Artery Surgery Affect Survival? Analysis of 1987–1992 Manitoba Administrative Data." *Annual Meeting of International Society of Technology Assessment in Health Care* 11 (1995): Abstract No. 215.

15 A. Morris, L. Roos, R. Brazauskas, and D. Bedard, "Managing Scarce Services: A Waiting List Approach to Cardiac Catheterization." *Medical Care* 28 (1990): 784–92.

16 C. D. Naylor, K. Sykora, S. B. Jaglal, and S. Jeffersons, "Waiting for Coronary Bypass Surgery: Population-Based Study of 8,517 Consecutive Patients in Ontario, Canada." *Lancet* 346 (1995): 1605–09.

17 J. L. Cox, J. G. Petrie, P. T. Pollak, and D. E. Johnstone, "Managed Delay for Coronary Artery Bypass Graft Surgery: The Experience at

One Canadian Center." *Journal of the American College of Cardiologists* 27 (1996): 1365–73.

18 M. Carrier, R. Pineault, N. Tremblay, and C. Pelletier, "Outcome of Rationing Access to Open Heart Surgery: Effect of the Wait for Elective Surgery on Patient Outcome." *Canadian Medical Association Journal* 149 (1993): 1117–22.

19 S. J. Bernstein, H. Rigter, and A. Meijler, "Waiting for Coronary Revascularization in the Netherlands." *Annual Meeting of International Society of Technology Assessment in Health Care* 11 (1995): Abstract No. 60.

20 M. J. Suttorp, J. H. Kingma, J. Vos, E. M. Koomen, J. G. Tijssen, and F. E. Vermeulen, et al, "Determinants for Early Mortality in Patients Awaiting Coronary Artery Bypass Graft Surgery: A Case-Control Study." *European Heart Journal* 13 (1992): 238–42.

21 A. Bengtson, T. Karlsson, A. Hjalmarson, and J. Herlitz, "Complications Prior to Revascularization among Patients Waiting for Coronary Artery Bypass Grafting and Percutaneous Transluminal Coronary Angioplasty." *European Heart Journal* 17 (1996): 1846–51.

22 M.L. Barer and S. Lewis, "Waiting for Health Care in Canada: Problems and Prospects," prepared for the Dialogue on Health Reform (2000).

23 B. Starfield, "Is US Health Really the Best in the World?" Commentary, *Journal of the American Medical Association*, 284(4) (2000): 483–85.

24 Victor Godinez, "Metro Hospitals Diverting Patients," *Dallas Morning News* (May 10, 2001). Report documents nationwide problem.

25 *More Money Would Put an End to Emergency Room Crunches*, Canadian Health Services Research Foundation Mythbusters Series No. 1 (Winter 2001).

26 It is often suggested that privately purchasing medical services would reduce the pressures on the public sector and allow for reduced waiting lists. This has certainly not occurred in the U.K. despite the option of buying private care, which is exercised by about 13 percent of the population. See W. Hutton, *New Life for Health: The Commission on the NHS* (London: Vintage, 2000).

27 C. Richmond, "NHS Waiting Lists Have Been a Boon for Private Medicine in the U.K.," *Canadian Medical Association Journal* 154 (1996): 378–81.

28 C. Tuohy, C. Flood, and M. Stabile, *How Does Private Finance Affect Public Health Care Systems? Marshalling the Evidence from OECD Systems* (Toronto: Canadian Health Economics Research Association, May 2001).

29 *A Parallel Private System Would Reduce Waiting Times in the Public System,* Canadian Health Services Research Foundation Mythbusters Series No. 2.

30 T. Besley, J. Hall, and I. Preston, "Private and Public Health Insurance in the UK," *European Economic Review* 42 (1998): 491–97.

31 Lewis and Sanmartin, "Managing Waiting Lists."

32 Ibid.

CHAPTER 5 ➤ Closer to Home and Out of Pocket: Shifting Sites of Care

1 This chapter draws heavily from the two papers commissioned by the Dialogue on Health Reform, which can be found on our Web site: http://www.utoronto.ca/hpme/dhr.

P. C. Coyte, "Home Care in Canada: Passing the Buck" (May 2000) and M. Anderson and K. Parent, "Care in the Home: Public Responsibility/Private Roles?" (June 2000).

2 Statistics Canada, Population estimates for 1996 and projection for the years 2001, 2006, 2011, and 2016. (March 3, 1999) http://www.statcan. ca/english/Pgdb/People/Population/demo23a.htm.

3 P. Baranek and P. C. Coyte, "Long-Term Care in Ontario: Home Care and Residential Care," Report for the College of Physicians and Surgeons of Ontario (May 1999).

4 Health and Welfare Canada, *Report on Home Care* (Ottawa: Federal/ Provincial Working Group on Home Care, 1990).

5 Health and Welfare Canada, *Canada Health Act, Revised Statutes of Canada* (1989).

6 P. Baranek, "Institutions and Interests on the Public/Private Mix, Long-Term Care Reform in Ontario: The Influence of Ideas," Ph.D. Thesis, University of Toronto (2000).

7 "Home Health Care: Only If You Can Afford It," *Globe and Mail* (December 6, 1999).

8 PriceWaterhouseCoopers Health Care Group, "Health Insider: An In Depth Research Report on Consumer Health Issues," Toronto, Survey No. 2 (November 1999).

9 "How Would You Pay For Home Care?" *Toronto Star,* November 27, 1999).

10 Coyte, "Passing the Buck"; Anderson and Parent, "Care in the Home."

11 Baranek and Coyte, "Long-Term Care in Ontario."

12 Health Services Utilization and Research Commission, "The Impact of Preventive Home Care and Seniors Housing on Health Outcomes," Summary Report No. 14 (May 2000).

13 P. C. Coyte and W. Young, "Reinvestment in and Use of Home Care Services," Institute for Clinical Evaluative Sciences, Technical Report No. 97-05-TR (November 1997).

14 P. C. Coyte, W. Young, and D. De Boer, "Home Care Report, Report to the Health Services Restructuring Commission" (April 1997).

15 Health Services Restructuring Commission, "Rebuilding Ontario's Health System: Interim Planning Guidelines and Implementation Strategies" (July 1997).

16 K. Parr, *The Cost Effectiveness of Home Care: A Literature Review* (Saskatoon, Saskatchewan: Health Services Utilization and Research Commission, March 1996).

17 Price Waterhouse, "Operational Review of the Ontario Home Care Program, Final Report" (1989).

18 Federal/Provincial/Territorial Working Group on Home Care, *A Working Group of the Federal/Provincial/Territorial Subcommittee on Long Term Care:* Report on Home Care (Ottawa: Health Services Promotion Branch, Health and Welfare Canada, 1990).

19 Marcus Hollander, "The Preventative and Maintenance Function of Home Care: An Empirical Analysis," paper presented to the Ninth Canadian Conference on Health Economics, University of Toronto, Toronto, Canada (May 25, 2001).

20 M. MacAdam, "Home Care: It's Time for a Canadian Model," *Healthcare Papers* 1 (4) (2000): 937.

21 A. Cueller and J. Weiner, "Can Social Insurance for Long-Term Care Work? The Experience of Germany," *Health Affairs*, 19(3) (2000): 8–25.

22 MacAdam, "Home Care."

23 K. Nagasawa, "Public Long-Term Care Insurance of the Elderly in Japan: Its Framework and Its Challenges," presentation to the Home Care Evaluation and Research Centre, University of Toronto (February 14, 2001).

24 J. Campbell and N. Ikegami, "Long-Term Care Insurance Comes to Japan," *Health Affairs* 19(3) (2000): 26–39.

25 National Forum on Health, *Canada Health Action: Building on the Legacy* (St. Foy, Quebec: Editions Multimondes 1997).

CHAPTER 6 ➤ The Future: Rigid, Resilient, or Retail Reform Choices

1 See K. Kenna, "First Lady Blasts U.S. Drug Prices," *Toronto Star*, (February 9, 2000).

2 D. Price, A. Pollock, and J. Shaoul, "How the World Trade Organisation Is Shaping Domestic Policies in Health Care," *Lancet* 354 (November 27, 1999): 1889–92.

3 B. Appleton, "International Agreements and National Health Plans: NAFTA," in D. Drache and T. Sullivan, eds., *Health Reform, Public Success Private Failure*, (London: Routledge, 1999).

4 S. Shrybman, "A Legal Opinion Concerning NAFTA Investment and Services Disciplines and Bill 11: Proposals by Alberta to Privatize the Delivery of Certain Health Services," legal opinion to the Canadian Union of Public Employees (March 2000).

5 B. Appleton, "NAFTA Investment Chapter Implications of Alberta Bill 11," legal opinion to the Canadian Health Coalition (April 10, 2000).

6 La commission d'étude sur les services de santé et les services sociaux: Les solutions emergents, Ministère de la Santé et des Services Sociaux (Quebec: Bibliothèque Legal du Quebec). http://www.msss.gouv. qc.ca.

7 "Caring for Medicare: Sustaining a Quality System, Final report of the Commission on Medicare in Saskatchewan" (2001), *Saskatchewan Health* (April, 2001) http://www.medicare-commission.com/finalreport. htm.

8 Tuohy, C., C. Flood, M. Stabile, "How Does Private Finance Affect Public Health Care Systems? Marshalling the Evidence from OECD Systems," Canadian Health Economics Research Association, Toronto, May, 2001.